OBSTETRICS AND GYNECOLOGY ADVANCES

SUCCEEDING IN MRCOG PART 2

A QUESTION BANK OF 400 EMQS AND SBAS

Obstetrics and Gynecology Advances

Additional books in this series can be found on Nova's website under the Series tab.

Additional e-books in this series can be found on Nova's website under the e-books tab.

OBSTETRICS AND GYNECOLOGY ADVANCES

SUCCEEDING IN MRCOG PART 2

A QUESTION BANK OF 400 EMQS AND SBAS

SHARMISTHA GUHA
PARIJAT BHATTACHARJEE
NUTAN MISHRA
AND
FRANCIS AYIM

nova publishers
New York

Library of Congress Cataloging-in-Publication Data

ISBN: 978-1-63485-407-8
Library of Congress Control Number: 2016941626

Published by Nova Science Publishers, Inc. † New York

CONTENTS

FOREWORD

The MRCOG Part 2 examination has evolved over recent years and now provides a more comprehensive assessment of both the theoretical, clinical and communication skills essential to the successful 21st century specialist.

My colleagues have worked tirelessly to produce an excellent EMQ and SBA Question book which will provide essential examination preparation for the aspiring specialist.

This examination preparation book will be as equally useful to those practicing in the United Kingdom and to those working abroad. The questions included are drawn from all modules in the curriculum and will provide a challenging but realistic test of the candidate's knowledge.

References and detailed explanations provide support for the candidates and will help them broaden their specialty knowledge. This will provide a sound foundation for success.

I hope you find this both challenging and helpful. I wish you well in your professional journey.

Mr Gregory H Ward
FRCOG
Consultant Obstetrician & Gynaecologist
Head of the London Specialty School of O&G
RCOG Examiner and Member of RCOG SBA Committee
Member, RCOG Specialty Education Advisory Committee

PREFACE

The MRCOG Part 2 Examination has gone through many changes in recent years. The focus has shifted to the assessment of clinical skills and applied clinical knowledge along with communication and patient safety. The Extended Matching Questions (EMQs) were introduced in 2006 and more recently the Single Best Answers (SBAs) in 2015. Our aim was to produce a comprehensive set of both types of questions covering all the modules of the MRCOG Part 2 syllabus (www.rcog.org.uk). A broad range of reading material has been used to develop the EMQs and SBAs including RCOG Greentop Guidelines, Scientific Impact Papers, Clinical Governance Papers and RCOG Consent Advice. In addition to the RCOG revision material we have included questions from The Obstetrician & Gynaecologist (TOG), NICE Guidelines, StratOG and recommended textbooks.

The authors have experience in MRCOG Examination Question writing and Sharmistha Guha has been a co-lead for the London SBA Writing Group for the RCOG. The questions have been written to the same standard as the RCOG question bank.

It is important to recognize that this book is not a text book and should not be used as the sole reading material for the examination. However, the questions will be especially useful in gaining valuable examination practice. An explanation has been provided for all of the questions along with references to aid in your preparation. We have included a reading guide to assist you and the questions have been written in the same format as in the examination.

This is the first book which combines a large number of both EMQs and SBAs and we believe it will prove an essential and important preparatory book for the Part 2. We hope you find it a valuable resource for your preparation.

Chapter 1

ALL ABOUT MRCOG PART 2

The Part 2 MRCOG examination has evolved over the years. Various formats have been used and question patterns have changed. Multiple-choice questions remained one of the mainstays of the examination but have been replaced by Single Best Answer Questions (SBAs) to better assess a candidate's judgment and clinical decision making in a given clinical scenario as opposed to simply assessing factual knowledge.

It is imperative that candidates are familiar with the types of different question formats and the correct way to assess and answer them. For overseas candidates, not familiar with the functioning of the NHS or the UK healthcare system, it is essential to acquaint themselves with the workings of the NHS.

There are 17 modules in the MRCOG syllabus, which will be tested in both the theoretical and clinical part of the examination. The details of the complete modules can be found at https://www.rcog.org.uk/en/careers-training/mrcog-exams/part-2-mrcog/syllabus/. The book covers all modules of the examination in both Obstetrics and Gynaecology and contains over 400 questions covering a wide variety of clinical scenarios and contexts. This is expected to give the candidates extensive practice in preparing for the examination. The examination pattern is as below:

Paper 1: 50 SBAs and 50 EMQs (3 hours)
Paper 2: 50 SBAs and 50 EMQs (3 hours).

There is 40% weightage to SBAs and 60% to EMQs in each paper and the minimum standard is determined by a complex standard setting process. Modified Angoff method is used for MRCOG Part 2 standard setting. More details can be found at https://www.rcog.org.uk/en/careers-training/mrcog-exams/mrcog-pass-mark/.

EMQ

Extended matching questions follow a definite structure. There are 10 to 14 *options* tabulated in alphabetical or numerical order. This is followed by a *stem* or instruction. This is the lead-in. It instructs the candidate what is expected of them. Then there is a list of about 5 – 8 questions which matches the numbers on the answer sheet.

On the answer sheet there are corresponding question numbers with 20 lozenges A to T, which corresponds to the options. Since there are only 10 – 14 options, all of the lozenges will not be used. There may be one or more than one answer which may be relevant but the candidate is expected to choose the one most appropriate in the context. There are no negative marks for wrong answers. However, if 2 or more lozenges are marked for a particular question, you don't get any marks for it.

SBA

Single Best Answer questions have a stem or *lead-in* statement that outlines the clinical scenario. This is followed by the instructions. A list of 5 *options* marked A-E (as represented in the Answer sheet) follow this stem. There may be more than one correct answer to a question but the *most appropriate* answer is to be chosen.

Details of the examination format can be found at

https://www.rcog.org.uk/en/careers-training/mrcog-exams/part-2-mrcog/format/

TIPS

We would like to reiterate some basic tips for success in the examination. Please read the question carefully and get an idea of what aspect of your knowledge is being tested. There is no hidden 'catch' in any of the questions. Therefore, please read between the lines.

Although shortage of time is not so much a factor in the current pattern of the examination, it is important to keep some time for cross checking your answers in the final answer sheet.

Lastly, it is important to thoroughly cover all the modules when you are preparing for the examination. It is important to know that all the domains and modules are tested in the MRCOG Part 2 examination and are mapped by the Blueprinting process.

We wish you all the best for your success.

Chapter 2

LIST OF READING MATERIAL

TEXTBOOKS

1) Chamberlain G. *Turnbulls Obstetrics* (3e). Churchill Livingstone; 2001.
2) Drife J, Magowan B. *Clinical Obstetrics and Gynaecology*. Saunders; 2004.
3) Luesley D, Baker P. *Obstetrics and Gynaecology: an evidence-based text for MRCOG*. Arnold; 2004.
4) Nelson-Piercy C. *Handbook of Obstetric Medicine*. Taylor and Francis; 2006.
5) Shaw R, Soutter WP and Stanton SL. *Gynaecology (3e)*.Churchill Livingstone; 2003.
6) MBRRACE-UK: Mothers and Babies: Reducing Risk through Audits and Confidential Enquiries across the UK

JOURNALS

1) The Obstetrician and Gynaecologist (TOG)
2) British Journal of Obstetrics & Gynaecologists (BJOG)

WEBSITES

1) Royal College of Obstetrics and Gynaecology (RCOG). https://www.rcog.org.uk/en/

2) National Institute for Health and Care Excellence
https://www.nice.org.uk/guidance?action=bytopic&o=7252
3) Cochrane Database of Pregnancy and Childbirth
http://pregnancy.cochrane.org

Chapter 3

EXTENDED MATCHING QUESTIONS (EMQS)

Options for Questions 1 – 5

A. Barrier Method	I. Medroxyprogesterone acetate 104mg
B. Combined oral Contraceptive with 30μg ethinylestradiol	J. Etonorgesterol 68mg
C. Combined oral contraceptive with 50μg ethinylestradiol	K. Etonorgesterol with barium 68mg
D. Levonorgesterol 1500mg	L. Desogesterol 75μg
E. Ullipristal acetate 5mg	M. Combined oral contraceptive with 20μg ethinylestradiol
F. Ullipristal acetate 30mg	N. Levonorgesterol 30μg
G. Depot medroxyprogesterone acetate 150mg	O. Levonorgesterol 3000mg
H. Noristerate 200mg	

Instructions

For the following case scenarios, please choose the single best form of contraception from the above list of options. Each option may be used once, more than once, or not at all.

1) A 27 year old woman recently returned from India and is on an enzyme inducing antituberculosis drug (not rifampicin) for the treatment of tuberculosis. She states she gets irregular bleeding with progesterone only contraception and wants short-term contraception.

2) A 38 year old woman with history of breast cancer diagnosed 7 years ago. She has remained disease free for 5 years
3) A 30 year old woman has come for emergency contraception as she had unprotected sexual intercourse 4 days ago.
4) A 42 year old lady complains of persistent irregular bleeding with Micronor. She is a chronic smoker and has a BMI of 37.
5) A 34 year old is 25 days postpartum. She is not breastfeeding and wants to start taking contraception pills. She does not want any other form of contraception.

Options for Questions 6 – 9

A. IV Augmentin 1.2gm 1 hour prior to procedure	G. Oral Augmentin 625mg TDS x 7 days
B. IV Augmentin 1.2gm after the procedure	A. Oral Metronidazole 400mg TDS x 7 days
C. PR Metronidazole 1gm	I. IV Ampicillin
D. IV Gentamycin	J. IV Augmentin + IV metronidazole at the time of procedure
E. IV Tazocin	K. IV Clindamycin prior to procedure
F. IV Cefuroxime 1.5gm + IV Metronidazole	L. No antibiotic

Instructions

For the following scenarios, please choose the single most appropriate antibiotic regime from the above list of options. Each option may be used once, more than once, or not at all.

6) A 34 year old patient is having elective caesarean section for breech
7) A 42 year old patient has delivered and sustained a 3rd degree tear. She is being taken to theatre
8) A 32 year old patient had manual removal of placenta and is now day 1 post delivery and is well.
9) An 18 year old is undergoing surgical termination of pregnancy.

Options for Questions 10 – 17

A. Colposcopy in 6 months	B. Radical trachealectomy
C. Colposcopy in 12 months	D. LLETZ
E. Cervical smear in 6 months	F. Cone Biopsy
G. HPV testing in 6 months	H. Colposcopy within 2 weeks
I. Cervical smear in 12 months	J. Colposcopy within 4 weeks
K. HPV testing in 12 months	L. Colposcopy within 6 weeks
M. Repeat smear in 3 months	N. Routine recall

Instructions

For the following scenario, please choose the single most appropriate management plan from the above list of options. Each option may be used once, more than once, or not at all.

10) A 27 year old woman had her second smear that came back as borderline. High Risk HPV test is positive
11) A 37 year old woman has low grade dyskaryosis and High Risk HPV Is negative
12) A 26 year old woman had her first smear which was moderate dyskaryosis
13) A 46 year old woman has 3 inadequate smear repeated 3 months apart
14) A 30 year old woman had LLETZ for CIN 3
15) A 34 year old woman had cone biopsy for CGIN 6 months ago. Test of cure is negative at present
16) A 55 year old woman had LLETZ for CIN3 and the deeper margins are not clear of CIN3.
17) A 45 year old had excisional treatment of microinvasive cancer FIGO stage Ia1. The excisional margins shows CIN

Options for Questions 18 – 23

A. Insert Levonorgestrol – releasing intrauterine system (LNG – IUS)	B. LNG – IUS for 6 months
C. Continuous oral progesterone therapy	D. Weight loss
E. Cyclical oral progesterone therapy	F. Repeat endometrial biopsy in 3 months

G. Total abdominal hysterectomy + Bilateral salpingo-oophorectomy	H. Repeat endometrial biopsy in 6 months
I. Total laparoscopic hysterectomy + Bilateral salpingo-oophorectomy	J. Discharge
K. Total laparoscopic hysterectomy + conservation of ovaries	L. Endometrial ablation
M. Continuous progesterone for 6 months	N. Progesterone + endometrial surveillance in 3 months

Instructions

For the following scenario, please choose the single most appropriate management plan from the above list of options. Each option may be used once, more than once, or not at all.

18) A 54 year old lady presents with postmenopausal bleeding. The pipelle biopsy shows endometrial hyperplasia without atypia. She declines to have a coil.
19) A 43 year old Para 2 lady has BMI of 46. She complains of menorrhagia and the pipelle biopsy shows endometrial hyperplasia without atypia. She had Mirena coil inserted 2 years ago, but the symptoms have recurred.
20) A 42 year old Para 3 woman is diagnosed with endometrial hyperplasia with atypia. She had oral progesterone therapy. Her follow up endometrial pipelle biopsy at 12 months shows endometrial hyperplasia without atypia.
21) A 49 year old lady complained of menorrhagia and was found to have endometrial hyperplasia without atypia 2 years ago. She had the Mirena coil at the time. She had 2 pipelle biopsies 6 months apart and they were normal.
22) A 39 year old nulliparous lady complains of menorrhagia. She is found to have endometrial hyperplasia with atypia. She wants to conceive soon.
23) A 56 year old lady is on tamoxifen and complains of postmenopausal bleeding. She is found to have multiple polyps on transvaginal scan and the endometrial biopsy shows endometrial hyperplasia without atypia.

Options for 24 – 26

A. Cervical preparation with 200 μg misoprostol	B. F. Oral opiates
C. Topical local anaesthetic to ectocervix	D. Intravenous anaesthetic
E. No cervical preparation	F. Cervical preparation with 400 μg misoprostol
G. Paracervical/ Intracervical block	H. Oral mifepristone
I. IV 0.25mg Fentanyl + 0.5mg Atropine + 2mg midazolam	J. No cervical anaesthetic

Instructions

For the following case scenario, please choose the single most appropriate preoperative plan for outpatient hysteroscopy from the above list of options. Each option may be used once, more than once, or not at all.

24) A 36 year old nulliparous lady complains of intermenstrual bleeding. She is booked for outpatient hysteroscopy. The transvaginal scan shows a normal uterine cavity
25) A 42 year old parous lady is found to have a 2cm endometrial polyp on ultrasound scan. She is scared of general anaesthetic.
26) A 52 year old is undergoing outpatient hysteroscopy to investigate Post Menopausal Bleeding. She has Grade 2 vaginal wall prolapse and needs tenaculum for grasping the cervix.

Options for Questions 27 – 31

A. Injury to Inferior epigastric artery	B. Injury to Phrenic nerve
C. Injury to Lateral cutaneous nerve	D. Injury to Obturator Nerve
E. Injury to Aorta	F. Injury to Genito femoral nerve
G. Injury to Internal iliac artery	H. Injury to Iliohypogastric nerve
I. Injury to Ureter	J. Injury to Pudendal nerve

Instructions

For the following scenario, please choose the single most appropriate complication from the above list of options. Each option may be used once, more than once, or not at all.

27) A 34 year old has undergone a laparoscopic ovarian cystectomy. While in recovery, she complains of a painful swelling in the left iliac fossa. On examination, she has a 6 cm swelling under the left port site.
28) A 64 year old woman with history of hysterectomy in the past has an anterior repair. She presents 3 weeks later with gradual onset severe pain in the left side of the abdomen. On examination, she has left loin tenderness.
29) A 54 years old woman complains of stress incontinence and has undergone a sling operation. She presents 6 weeks later with complains of numbness in her inner thigh and difficulty in adduction of the thigh.
30) A 65 year old woman undergoes laparotomy and debulking surgery for ovarian mass. She presents 5 weeks later with paresthesia and pain radiating down the anterior and postero-lateral aspect of the thigh towards the knee.
31) A 69 year old lady had a history of hysterectomy 12 years ago. She complains of vault prolapse and has a sacrospinous fixation. On her follow up visit, she complains of pain in the perineum mainly on sitting down.

Options for Questions 32 – 37

A. BRCA 1 Gene Mutation	B. Peutz-Jegher's Syndrome
C. BRCA 2 Gene Mutation	D. Li-Fraumeni Syndrome
E. Werner Syndrome	F. Lynch Syndrome
G. Cowden Syndrome	H. Multiple Endocrine Neoplasia Type 1
I. Bannayan-Riley-Ruvalcaba Syndrome	J. Multiple Endocrine Neoplasia Type 2

Instructions

For the following scenario, please choose the single most appropriate genetic syndrome from the above list of options. Each option may be used once, more than once, or not at all.

32) A 45 year old lady has 63% risk of ovarian cancer and 85% risk of breast cancer by age 70.
33) A 32 year old lady is diagnosed with this syndrome, which puts her at high risk of having synchronous endometrial cancer with ovarian cancer.
34) A 30 year old woman has 27% risk of ovarian cancer and 84% risk of breast cancer.
35) A 10 year old girl is found to have germline mutation in the tumour suppressor gene PTEN.
36) A 43 year old woman is found to have an autosomal dominant gastrointestinal polyposis disorder
37) A 19 year old young woman is found to have germline TP53 mutation

Options for Questions 38 – 41

A. Pfannesteil Incision	B. Mouchel Incision
C. Joel – Cohen Incision	D. Midline Incision
E. Maylard Incision	F. Paramedian Incision
G. Küstner incision	H. Rockey- Davis Incision
I. Cherney Incision	J. Gridiron Incision of McBurney

Instructions

For the following scenario, please choose the single most appropriate incision from the above list of options. Each option may be used once, more than once, or not at all.

38) A 34 year old lady is having caesarean section and she has a straight transverse incision on the skin 3cm below the anterior superior iliac spine. The subcutaneous tissue and fascia are opened in the midline by blunt dissection.

39) A 49 year old lady is having a total abdominal hysterectomy for a normal sized uterus. She had 4 caesarean sections in the past. She has an incision in which all layers of the abdominal wall are incised transversely 6 cm above the symphysis pubis.

40) A 56 year old lady is having oophorectomy for a 24 cm dermoid ovarian cyst.

41) A 20 year old lady is having an open appendectomy.

Options for Questions 42 – 47

A.	Vault Hematoma	B.	G. Deep Vein Thrombosis
C.	Vesico-vaginal fistula	D.	H. Ureteric Injury
E.	Disseminated Intravascular Coagulopathy	F.	I. Bladder Injury
G.	Sepsis	H.	J. Pulmonary Embolism
I.	Lymphorrhoea	J.	K. Bowel Injury
K.	Paralytic Ileus	L.	L. Pneumothorax

Instructions

For the following scenario, please choose the single most appropriate postoperative complication from the above list of options. Each option may be used once, more than once, or not at all.

42) A 34 year old lady had a surgical termination of pregnancy. She presents 2 days later with pyrexia and rigors. She is found to have tachypnea, tachycardia and a temperature of 39°C on initial assessment

43) A 56 year old lady has total abdominal hysterectomy. She has history of atrial fibrillation and is on warfarin. She present 1 week later with pain in lower abdomen and vaginal discharge.

44) A 34 year old lady has laparoscopic adhesiolysis of bowel adhesions and treatment to endometriosis. She complains of abdominal pain postoperatively and vomiting. On examination, the abdomen is distended and the bowel sounds are tympanic.

45) A 47 year old lady has laparoscopic assisted vaginal hysterectomy. She presents with right-sided abdominal pain. A CT Scan shows a 3cm encysted space on the right pelvic side wall with clear fluid.

46) A 60 year old lady has laparoscopic hysterectomy and para aortic lymphadenectomy for endometrial cancer. She presents 10 days later with history of blood stained fluid per vaginum. The biochemical profile of the fluid is same as her serum profile.

47) A 36 year old lady had caesarean section 4 months ago. She presents with history of leaking clear fluid at all times. She has to wear pad at all times.

Options for Questions 48 – 51

A. 71%	B. 86%
C. 74%	D. I. 4.09
E. 69%	F. J. 5.07
G. 82%	H. 0.40
I. 87%	J. 6.0
K. 0.34	L. 0.23
M. 5.5	N. 84%

Instructions

A diagnostic test is applied to 1500 women to assess susceptibility to IUGR. The prevalence of IUGR is 3%.

	IUGR Present	IUGR Absent
Test Positive	50	200
Test Negative	20	1230

For the above scenario, please choose the single most appropriate answer from the above list of options. Each option may be used once, more than once, or not at all.

48) Find out the sensitivity of the diagnostic test
49) Find out the specificity of the diagnostic test
50) Find out the positive likelihood ratio
51) Find out the negative likelihood ratio

Options for Questions 52 – 57

A. Tubal cannulation	B. Gonadotrophin & IUI
C. Salpingotomy	D. IUI
E. Salpingectomy & IVF	F. Operative hysteroscopy
G. IVF/ICSI	H. Ablation/Excision of endometriosis & adhesiolysis
I. Natural cycle IVF	J. Excision of rectal/ureteric endometriotic nodule & adhesiolysis +/- G.I. surgeon/Urology involvement

Instructions

For each case scenario described below, choose the single most appropriate management plan from the above list of options. Each option may be used once, more than once, or not at all.

52) A 36 year old woman presents with secondary subfertility. A proximal tubal occlusion is noted on HSG.
53) A 32 year old woman presents with primary subfertility for 2 years. She has left hydrosalpinx on pelvic ultrasound. She also has multiple subserous and intramural fibroids.
54) A 35 year old woman presents with primary subfertility of 3 years duration and amenorrhoea of 6 months. The pelvic ultrasound and HSG suggests intrauterine adhesions.
55) A 37 year old lady with ASA Stage 4 endometriosis diagnosed at Laparoscopy presents with primary subfertility.
56) A young couple where all investigations are normal but the husband is HIV positive.
57) A 35 year old lady presents with primary subfertility. They are trying to conceive for a year having regular unprotected intercourse. The partner's semen analysis is normal. Her hormonal profile, ultrasound scan of pelvis and tubal patency test are all normal. Her luteal phase progesterone is ovulatory.

Options for Questions 58 – 63

A. Clomiphene	B. IVF/ICSI
C. Gonadotrophins (incl. LH/HCG)	D. IUI with partner or donor sperm
E. GnRH pulsatile	F. IUI with Gonadotrophin stimulation
G. Metformin	H. Anastrozole/Letrozole
I. Laparoscopic ovarian drilling	J. Natural cycle IVF
K. Bromocriptine/Cabergoline	L. Growth hormone/DHEAS & IVF

Instructions

For each case described below, choose the single most likely management plan from the above list of options. Each option may be used once, more than once, or not at all.

58) An athlete practicing intensely for the marathon presents with oligomenorrhoea and primary subfertility.
59) A 38year old lady with BMI of 32 presents in a secondary centre with secondary subfertility and oligomenorrhoea. Husband's semen and tubal patency test are normal. She is not eligible for IVF in the NHS and unable to afford privately. She had 6 months of clomiphene at increasing dosage but cycles were anovulatory.
60) A 30 year old woman with a normal BMI presents to the fertility clinic with oligomenorrhoea and the following hormonal profile: Luteal phase progesterone – anovulatory; LH: 7 mu/l; FSH 6 mu/l; Prolactin: 2000 mu/l. The results are consistent on repeat testing. She is not on any medications. Thyroid function test and testosterone levels are normal.
61) A 30year old woman with Type 2 diabetes and a BMI of 32 presents with oligomenorrhoea and anovulatory subfertility.
62) A 41year old woman is seen in the fertility clinic with her partner trying to conceive for 2 years. Her AMH is 18pmol/l. They are diagnosed to have unexplained subfertility.
63) A lesbian couple with normal investigations presents to fertility clinic trying to conceive

Options for Questions 64 – 68

A.	Low dose Aspirin	B.	Serial Cervical length ultrasound scan
C.	Prednisolone	D.	HCG
E.	Low molecular weight Heparin	F.	Metformin
G.	Hysteroscopic resection	H.	Intravenous immunoglobulin
I.	Cervical cerclage	J.	Reassurance
K.	Progesterone pessary	L.	Low dose Aspirin & LMW Heparin

Instructions

For each case scenario of recurrent/2nd trimester miscarriage described below, choose the single most likely management plan from the above list of options. Each option may be used once, more than once, or not at all.

64) A 28 year old lady presents at 10 weeks gestation with vaginal spotting. She gives history of two first trimester miscarriages and a second trimester miscarriage at 18 weeks suspected to be due to cervical weakness. Investigations were normal.
65) A 25 year old woman investigated for recurrent 1st trimester miscarriages, is found to have high titres of anticardiolipin antibodies.
66) A 32 year old woman being investigated for recurrent 1st trimester miscarriages. She has a BMI of 34 and a family history of Type 2 diabetes. She has been diagnosed to have PCOS. No other cause has been found.
67) A 25 year old woman had investigations abroad for recurrent 1st trimester miscarriages. All investigations are normal except uterine Natural Killer cells, which is positive.
68) A 32 year old lady has been investigated for recurrent first trimester miscarriages. A luteal phase defect has been the working diagnosis. She is now pregnant and it is a natural conception.

Options for Questions 69 – 73

A.	Mifepristone & Misoprostol	B.	Ergometrine
C.	Misoprostol	D.	Paracetamol
E.	NSAID	F.	Azithromycin
G.	Oxytocin	H.	Metronidazole
I.	Tranexamic acid	J.	Doxycycline

Instructions

For each case described below, choose the single most likely drug management from the above list of options. Each option may be used once, more than once, or not at all.

69) A 32 year old woman presents with mild vaginal bleeding. TV scan diagnoses missed miscarriage at 9 weeks gestation. She opts for medical management of her miscarriage.
70) A 36 year old woman is having a Termination of pregnancy at 12 weeks gestation following diagnosis of Trisomy 21 on CVS. She opts for medical management.
71) A 16 year old girl is having surgical termination of pregnancy at 7 weeks gestation. She has had endocervical swab that was negative for chlamydia. She is being given prophylactic medication at the time of the procedure.
72) A 25 year old woman just had a surgical termination of pregnancy at 9 weeks gestation. Prophylactic antibiotics have been prescribed. She is keen to take some analgesics.
73) A 32 year old woman is having moderate bleeding while undergoing surgical evacuation of a molar pregnancy of 12 weeks gestation. Anaesthetist is concerned and wants to give her some medication to decrease the bleeding.

Options for Questions 74 – 76

A. Cornual ectopic pregnancy	B. Missed miscarriage
C. Interstitial ectopic pregnancy	D. Ovarian ectopic pregnancy
E. Heterotopic pregnancy	F. Complete molar pregnancy
G. Caesarean scar ectopic	H. Incomplete miscarriage
I. Cervical ectopic pregnancy	J. Partial molar pregnancy
K. Abdominal pregnancy	L. Dichorionic twin pregnancy

Instructions

For each case described below, choose the single most likely diagnosis based on ultrasound scan findings from the above list of options. Each option may be used once, more than once, or not at all.

74) A 27 year old woman presents to Early pregnancy unit with moderate abdominal cramps and mild vaginal bleeding. She conceived through IVF. On transvaginal ultrasound scan, in the coronal plane of the uterus a thin line of the endometrium is seen and ends at the periphery of a hyperechogenic circular area seen with a thin rim of myometrium around.

75) A 33 year old lady presents to Early pregnancy unit with history of heavy vaginal bleeding. No product of conception is seen on speculum examination. On ultrasound scan, the sac is seen below the internal cervical os and the cervix is barrel shaped.

76) A 37 year old lady presents to Early Pregnancy unit with pain in right iliac fossa. She had IUI and clomid induction. She previously had a caesarean section. On ultrasound scan, a gestational sac with a fetal pole measuring 6mm is seen eccentrically placed in the endometrial cavity. The corpus luteum is on the right. There is a large amount of echogenic fluid in the POD and the right adnexa.

Options for Questions 77 – 81

A. Oxybutinin	F. Mirabegron
B. Tolteratidine	G. A. Transdermal oxybutinin
C. Duloxetine	H. B. Vaginal oestrogen
D. Imipramine	I. C. Bethanecol
E. Desmopressin	J. D. Oral HRT

Instructions

For each case described below, choose the single most likely drug management from the above list of options. Each option may be used once, more than once, or not at all.

77) A 50 year old lady with urgency, frequency and intractable nocturia
78) A 65 year old lady who does not want surgery for Stress Urinary Incontinence (SUI)
79) A 60 year old lady with poor bladder contractility
80) An 85 year old frail lady with Overactive Bladder (OAB)
81) A 60 year old lady in whom Oxybutinin, Tolteradine or Darifenacin tablets are ineffective

Options for questions 82 – 87

A.	Pelvic Floor Exercise	F.	Laparoscopic sacrocolpopexy
B.	Pessary	G.	Ilio-coccygeal fixation
C.	High uterosacral ligament suspension	H.	Vaginal mesh kits
D.	Colpocleisis	I.	McCall culdoplasty
E.	Abdominal sacrocolpoplexy	J.	Sacrospinous fixation

Instructions

For each case described below, choose the single most likely management plan from the above list of options. Each option may be used once, more than once, or not at all.

82) An 80 year old lady is suffering from vaginal vault prolapse for 14 years. She has been using pessaries for a long time but has been suffering from bleeding, ulceration and intractable pain and discomfort.

83) A 56 year old woman is worried about sexual dysfunction following surgery for vault prolapse.

84) A 60 year old woman has recurrence of vault prolapse following previous surgery for the same indication.

85) During vaginal hysterectomy on a 62 year old woman with utero vaginal prolapse, the vaginal vault is found to be at the introitus.

86) A 56 year old woman is having vaginal hysterectomy for utero vaginal prolapse. She is keen to have additional procedure to prevent vault prolapse in the future.

87) A 78 year old woman has stage 4 prolapse. She has multiple co-morbidities.

Options for Questions 88 – 91

A.	Inform parents	F. Refer for termination of pregnancy
B.	Inform school	G. Give contraception
C.	Inform police	H. Get consent from parent
D.	Inform social worker	I. Involve paediatricians
E.	Inform partner	J. Refer to Genitourinary Medicine clinic

Instructions

For each case described below, choose the single most appropriate step from the above list of options. Each option may be used once, more than once, or not at all.

88) You see a 14 ycar old in the family planning clinic. She lives with her parents but has not told her parents that she is 8 weeks pregnant which is unplanned and unwanted.
89) A 14 year old girl requesting termination of pregnancy but does not want her boyfriend or parents to know.
90) A 14 year old girl who is sexually active but does not want her parents to know requests contraception. On examination you notice possible bruises or rash that you are unsure about
91) A 16 year old girl who lives in a care home presents frequently to the family planning clinic requesting emergency contraception. She is now pregnant and requesting termination of pregnancy. On examination multiple bruises are noted on her body that she explains are due to fall.

Options for Questions 92 – 94

A. IM ceftriaxone 500 mg, oral metronidazole 400 mg BD & Doxycycline 100 mg BD x14 days	B. Clindamycin IV + Gentamycin IV then oral clindamycin or doxycycline or metronidazole
C. Ofloxacin 400 mg BD + Metronidazole 400 mg BD x 14 days	D. Ofloxacin IV + Metronidazole IV
E. Ceftriaxone500 mg IM, then Azithromycin 1g/week x 2 weeks	F. Laparoscopic drainage of pelvic abscess, salpingectomy & division of perihepatic adhesions
G. Moxifloxacin 400 mg OD x14 days	H. Ultrasound guided drainage of pelvic abscess
I. Ceftriaxone 2 g IV OD + IV/ PO Doxycycline 100 mg BD x14 days + Metronidazole 400 mg BD x14 days	J. Laparoscopic salpingo oophorectomy

Instructions

For each case described below, choose the single most likely management plan from the above list of options. Each option may be used once, more than once, or not at all.

92) A 15 year old girl presenting with negative pregnancy test and generalised lower abdominal pain is feeling feverish and unwell with a temperature of 37.6° C. She gives history of multiple sexual partners.
93) A 25 year old woman recently returned from holiday abroad, presents with signs and symptoms of PID.
94) A 22 year old woman had severe PID including lower abdominal and right upper quadrant pain. She had 48 hours of IV antibiotics in the hospital. But she is still pyrexial and unwell. Transvaginal ultrasound shows bilateral tuboovarian abscesses

Options for Questions 95 – 100

A. Candida	B. Herpes Simplex Virus
C. Bacterial vaginosis	D. Human Papilloma Virus
E. Trichomonas vaginalis	F. Actinomyces
G. Chlamydia	H. Staphylococcus Aureus
I. Gonococci	J. Group B Streptococcus

Instructions

For each case described below, choose the single most likely organism from the above list of options. Each option may be used once, more than once, or not at all.

95) A 23 year old woman had recurrent visits to GP with intermenstrual bleeding while being on Combined Oral Contraceptive pills. She had been treated repeatedly for Urinary Tract Infection though urine cultures were always negative.
96) A 25 year old woman is referred because of low-grade smear abnormality and contact bleeding while having smear. She gives history of postcoital bleeding.

97) A 35 year old lady presents with severe PID following TOP that was not covered by antibiotics. Her cervical smear report 6 weeks ago shows ‘clue cells.’

98) An 18 year old presenting with retention of urine and non-specific lower abdominal pain and vaginal discharge with lymphadenopathy.

99) A 32 year old woman who uses tampons for her heavy periods is brought to A&E with pyrexia, hypotension and an erythematous rash. Blood cultures are negative.

100) A 30 year old woman who uses Copper Intrauterine device for contraception is being treated for Pelvic Inflammatory Disease. However, she is not responding to antibiotics in spite of changing the regime. Cervical smear report had mentioned the presence of an organism six months ago but she was asymptomatic then and did not have any treatment.

Options for Questions 101 – 103

A	Atrophic Vaginitis	F	Dysfunctional Uterine Bleeding
B	Cervical Cancer	G	Endometrial Cancer
C	Cervical Ectropion	H	Endometrial Polyp
D	Cervical Polyp	I	Endometrial Hyperplasia
E	Cervical Intraepithelial Neoplasia	J	Fibroid Uterus
		K	Vulval Intraepithelial Neoplasia

Instructions

For each case described below, choose the single most likely diagnosis from the above list of options. Each option may be used once, more than once, or not at all.

101) A 54 year-old woman complains of postcoital bleeding. She has regular periods and does not have any significant gynaecological history. She has spotting after every episode of intercourse. Her last cervical smear was 3 months ago and was normal.

102) A 78 year-old woman is referred to rapid access gynaecology clinic with 1 episode of postmenopausal bleeding. The ultrasound scan is normal and shows an endometrial thickness of 2.5 mm. The pipelle biopsy is normal.

103) A 35 year-old woman presents with foul smelling discharge and irregular bleeding for 4 months. She gives history of passing small foul smelling lumps and has bleeding after every episode of intercourse and irregularly almost every day. She has not had any cervical smears in the past.

Options for Questions 104 – 106

A. Amniocentesis	F. Oral Glucose Tolerance Test
B. Chorionic Villous Sampling	G. Renal Ultrasound
C. Fetal Anomaly Scan	H. Serial Growth scan
D. Hb Electrophoresis	I. Urine Culture
E. Hepatic Serology	J. Urinary Protein/Creatinine Ratio

Instructions

For each case described below, choose the single most likely investigation from the above list of options. Each option may be used once, more than once, or not at all.

104) A 32-year old primiparous woman referred by her community midwife with blood pressure of 145/95mmHg with 1+ of protein on urinalysis. She had frontal headache and visual disturbance earlier today. Her booking blood pressure was 110/60mmHg.

105) A 35 year old primiparous woman is referred to Antenatal Clinic with a BMI of 39. She is currently 27 weeks pregnant with no other risk factors and has been well so far.

106) A 33 year old Asian woman at 33 weeks gestation presented to her GP with itching of palms and soles. Liver Function tests done by GP showed raised ALT. She comes to Antenatal Clinic and continues to itch.

Options for Questions 107 - 109

A. Placental praevia	F. Cervical cancer
B. Placental abruption	G. Retained Placenta
C. Vasa Praevia	H. Uterine rupture
D. Succenturiate Lobe	I. Thrombocytopaenia
E. Cervical Ectropion	J. Placenta Accreta

Instructions

For each case described below, choose the single most likely diagnosis from the above list of options. Each option may be used once, more than once, or not at all.

107) A 34-year-old woman presents to labour ward with contractions and spontaneous rupture of membranes with vaginal bleeding. On exmination abdomen is soft in between contractions CTG is as follows:

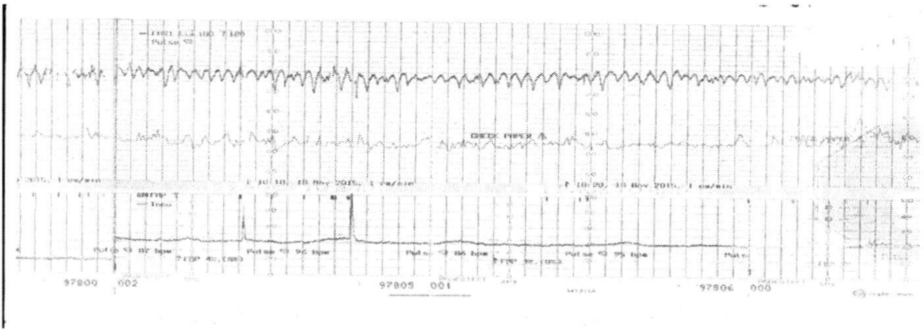

108) A 26-year-old woman presents to labour ward at 34 weeks with postcoital bleeding. Her recent smear was normal. The CTG on admission is as follows:

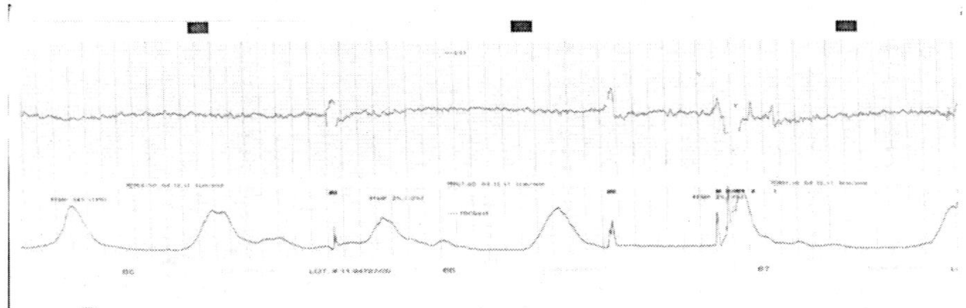

109) A 40-year-old woman in her second pregnancy presents to labour ward with abdominal pain. She is contracting 3 in 10. She had a

caesarean section in the first pregnancy for breech. The CTG on admission is as follows:

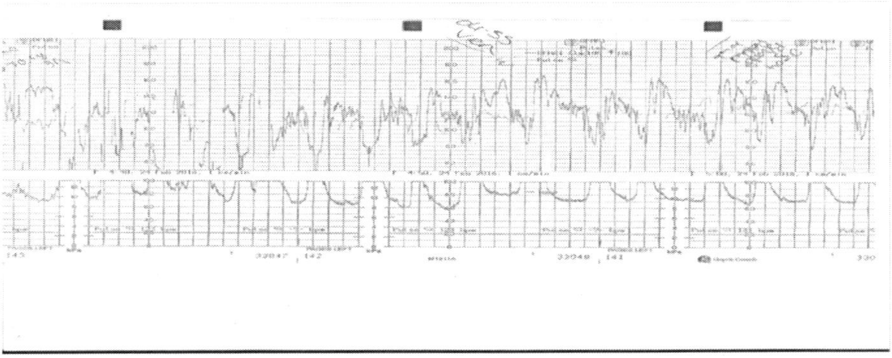

Options for Questions 110- 112

A. Myocardial infarction	F. Cardiomyopathy
B. Pulmonary Infarction	G. Aortic dissection
C. Pneumothorax	H. Pulmonary Embolism
D. Amniotic fluid embolism	I. Aortic rupture
E. Pericarditis	J. Acute pancreatitis

Instructions

For each case described below, choose the single most likely management plan from the above list of options. Each option may be used once, more than once, or not at all.

110) A 39-year-old woman who is 8 weeks postpartum started complaining of severe chest pain radiating to her left arm and then collapsed at home. Her husband called an ambulance and brought her to accident and emergency.

111) A 42-year-old woman with a BMI of 39 in her 4th pregnancy presented to her GP with chest tightness and breathlessness.

112) A 35-year-old woman was in labour in her first pregnancy. She had made slow progress and had been on syntocinon for the last 12 hours. She was having an emergency caesarean section for failure to progress when she suddenly collapsed on the table.

Options for Questions 113-115

A. Cytomegalovirus	F. HepatitisB
B. Herpes simplex	G. Chicken pox
C. Toxoplasmosis	H. Hepatitis A
D. Rubella	I. Gonorrhoea
E. Syphilis	J. Trichomonas

Instructions

For each case described below, choose the single most likely diagnosis from the above list of options. Each option may be used once, more than once, or not at all.

113) A 39-year-old woman is 16 weeks pregnant and is diagnosed with an infectious disease. She has been told that the infection can be transmitted to the baby at any stage of pregnancy if untreated.

114) A 35-year-old woman in her second pregnancy has been told that her infection can cause preterm birth and affect the baby's eyes at birth.

115) A 25-year-old woman at 20 weeks gestation is told that her infection can cause preterm birth but has very little other effect on the baby.

Options for Questions 116-118

A. Genital Herpes	F. Donovanosis
B. Herpes Zoster	G. Amoebiasis
C. Chancroid	H. Candidiasis
D. Syphilis	I. Bacterial vaginosis
E. Lymphogranuloma venereum	J. Trichomoniasis

Instructions

For each case described below, choose the single most likely diagnosis plan from the above list of options. Each option may be used once, more than once, or not at all.

116) A 27-year-old woman presents to her GP with vaginal discharge, dysuria and vulval irritation. Examination of the vulva shows purulent frothy malodorous discharge and punctate haemorrhage on the cervix.

117) A 44-year-old woman presents to her GP with itching and burning of her vulva and difficulty in passing urine. On examination the vulva is erythematous and swollen and a curdy white discharge is present

118) A 25-year-old woman presents to her GP with vulval irritation and finding difficulty in passing urine. On examination there are vesicles around the introitus.

Options for Questions 119 -121

A. Endometriosis	F. Nerve Entrapment
B. Ruptured ovarian cyst	G. Inflammatory bowel syndrome
C. Pelvic inflammatory disease	H. Fibroid degeneration
D. Appendicitis	I. Muscular pain
E. Ademomyosis	J. Interstitial Cystitis
	K. Diverticulitis

Instructions

For each case described below, choose the single most likely diagnosis from the above list of options. Each option may be used once, more than once, or not at all.

119) A 21-year-old woman presented with chronic pelvic pain, dymenorrhoea, dyspareunia and cyclical intestinal symptoms.

120) A 25-year-old woman presented with chronic pelvic pain and abdominal bloating that has no relationship with her periods and improves on defaecation.

121) A 35-year-old woman had a caesarean section 3 months ago and complains of localized pain on the right side of lower abdomen for the last 3 months. The examination of her abdomen is normal.

Options for Questions 122 –124

A Serum prolactin	G Progesterone challenge
B Laparoscopy	H Testosterone levels
C Karyotyping	I Thyroid function test
D Hysteroscopy	J Renal scan
E β HCG	K CT scan of head
F Reassurance & review	L Transvaginal USS

Instructions

For each case described below, choose the single most likely further investigation from the above list of options. Each option may be used once, more than once, or not at all.

122) A 27-year-old woman had menarche at the age of thirteen and regular periods. She has been on the oral contraceptive pill for the last 10 years and stopped the pill four months ago. She has been amenorrheric since stopping the pill. Pregnancy test is negative.

123) A 34 -year old woman presents with secondary amenorrhea for the last one year. Her investigations show a raised FSH and LH levels.

124) A 25-year-old woman presents with amenorrhoea for the last year. She has had regular periods before that. She had incidental finding on CT Scan of the head of 2.5 cm mass compressing the optic chiasma.

Options for Questions 125–128

A. Combined oral contraceptives	H. TAH +BSO
B. Danazol	I. Myomectomy
C. NSAIDs	J. Tranexamic acid
D. Antifibrinolytic	K. TAH
E. Endometrial ablation	L. TLH
F. Oral progestogens	M. TLH +BSO
G. IUD/ LNG-IUS	N. Ethamsylate

Instructions

For each case described below, choose the single most likely management plan from the above list of options. Each option may be used once, more than once, or not at all.

125) A 35-year old Para 2 woman presents with heavy menstrual bleeding. Her cycles are regular. On examination she has a normal size uterus. She had a trial of NSAIDs and tranexamic acid and she has family history of thromboembolism.

126) A 24 -year-old nulliparous woman presents with severe hirsutism. She also gives history of weight gain and irregular periods.

127) A 43-year-old woman has menorrhagia for last two years. She has completed her family and had a trial of Mirena coil which has not helped. On ultrasound scan she has 3 intramural fibroids measuring 2 X 2.5 cm. The uterus measured 8 x 6 x 5cm and the endometrial thickness is 6 mm.

128) A 44-year-old woman presents with severe menorrhagia for last 4 years. On ultra sound scan the uterus was 12 x10 x8cm endometrial thickness 8mm. She has tried Mirena IUS that has not been effective. She has severe premenstrual symptoms. Her BMI is 37.

Options for Questions 129–131

A Cognitive behavioural therapy	G Hysterectomy & bilateral salphingo-opherectomy
B Complementary therapy	H Hysterectomy
C Antidepressants	I Referral to Psychiatrist
D Estrogen	J Progesterone
E Oral contraceptive pill	K SSRI high dose
F GNRH analogues with add back HRT	L SSRI low dose

Instructions

For each case described below, choose the single most likely management plan from the above list of options. Each option may be used once, more than once, or not at all.

129) A 44-year-old woman is bothered by premenstrual symptoms a week before her periods. She has breast tenderness, bloatedness and headache. She has family history of venous thromboembolism.

130) A 42-year-old woman feels depressed, anxious, tense and has mood swings a week before her periods. She eats healthily and regularly exercises. She does not like any medication.

131) A 45 year-old woman gives history of getting violent three days before her periods. She has also been seen by the psychiatrist and tried hormonal therapy and SSRI.

Options for Questions 132 – 134

A. Azithromycin 1g	G. Benzyl penicillin
B. Ceftriaxone	H. Erythromycin
C. Metronidazole 400tds	I. Amoxycillin
D. Acyclovir 400mg BD	J. Ceftriaxone plus azithromycin
E. Acyclovir 400mg TDS	K. Clindamycin
F. Doxycycline	

Instructions

For each case described below, choose the single most likely drug treatment from the above list of options. Each option may be used once, more than once, or not at all.

132) A 34-year-old Para one woman at 15 weeks gestation was referred to your antenatal clinic as her booking blood showed a positive serology for Syphilis.

133) A 21-year-old woman presented to GUM clinic with excessive vaginal discharge and swab results confirmed Chlamydia. She was also found to be pregnant on urine pregnancy test.

134) A 36-year-old woman presents to your antenatal clinic with Herpes simplex lesions on her vulva. She is 37 weeks pregnant and had similar episodes in the past.

Options for Questions 135 – 138

A Mayer Rokitansky Küster Hauser Syndrome	F Unicornuate uterus
B Imperforate Hymen	G Bicornuate uterus
C Transvaginal septum	H Arcuate uterus
D Longitudinal vaginal septum	I Uterus Didelphus
E Rudimentary Horn	J Vaginal agenesis

Instructions

For each case described below, choose the single most likely diagnosis from the above list of options. Each option may be used once, more than once, or not at all.

135) A 27-year-old pregnant woman presented to A&E at 18 weeks gestation with severe abdominal pain. While waiting in A&E she collapsed and her blood pressure was 80/40mmHg with pulse of 120 bpm.

136) An 18-year-old woman presented to the gynaecology clinic with primary amenorrhoea. On examination, she has normal development of secondary sexual characteristics and cyclical mood swings. On vaginal examination a cervix is not palpable.

137) A 15-year-old girl presents to GP with cyclical abdominal pain and discomfort. On examination she has a palpable mass per abdomen. On inspection of vulva there is a pink bulging membrane.

138) A 15-year-old girl presents to A&E with abdominal pain and discomfort and has been unable to pass urine for the last 12 hours. On examination she has a palpable mass per abdomen. Inspection of vulva reveals a membrane that is blue in appearance.

Options for Questions 139 – 141

A. Topical oestrogen	G. SSRI
B. Acupuncture	H. SNRI
C. Clonidine	I. Gabapentin
D. Vitamins	J. Soya
E. Replens MD™	K. Transdermal Progesterone
F. St Johns Wort	L. DHEA

Instructions

For each case described below, choose the single most likely treatment from the above list of options. Each option may be used once, more than once, or not at all.

139) A 55-year-old woman with recent history of breast cancer has severe vasomotor symptoms she is on Tamoxifen.

140) A 55-year-old woman with recent history of oestrogen receptor negative breast cancer presents to the gynaecology clinic with severe vasomotor symptoms.

141) A 45- year -old woman with history of oestrogen receptor positive breast cancer has superficial dyspareunia due to vaginal dryness. She is on tamoxifen.

Options for Questions 142 – 144

A. Packed blood cell	F. Crystalloid
B. Cell salvage	G. Colloid
C. Cryo precipitate	H. Platelets
D. FFP	I. Recombinant factor VIIa
E. Anti D	J. Fibrinogen concentrate

Instructions

For each case described below, choose the single most likely management plan from the above list of options. Each option may be used once, more than once, or not at all.

142) A 44-year-old Para 4 had a normal vaginal delivery in the birth centre 20 minutes ago and has retained placenta, which was removed with gentle cord traction, but she continues to bleed and the estimated blood loss is now 2500ml. The fourth unit of red cell is running. The uterus now feels firm.

143) A 44-year-old Para 4 had a normal vaginal delivery in the birth centre 20 minutes ago and has a retained placenta that was removed with gentle cord traction but she continues to bleed and the estimated blood loss is now 2500ml. The fourth unit of red

cell is running. She continues to bleed and fibrinogen level is 0.8 gm/l

144) A 35 year old primiparous woman has severe preeclampsia and needs an emergency caesarean section. The anaesthetist refuses regional anaesthesia due to her blood results.

Options for Questions 145 – 147

A Vaginal examination	F Speculum examination (Sims)
B Breast examination	G High vaginal swab
C Rectal examination	I Endocervical swab
D Speculum examination (Cuscoes)	J Endocervical + rectal
E Abdominal examination	K Low vaginal swab

Instructions

For each case described below, choose the single most likely management plan from the above list of options. Each option may be used once, more than once, or not at all.

145) A 30-year-old lady presents to the gynaecology clinic with chronic pelvic pain, severe dysmenorrhoea and heavy menstrual bleeding. Ultrasound is normal, she has never been sexually active.

146) A 24-year-old woman presents to labour ward 6 days postnatal with vaginal discharge after delivering a preterm baby. Baby is admitted to Neonatal Unit and has problems with its eye.

147) A 54 -year-old Para 5 woman presents to gynaecology clinic with urgency and urge incontinence.

Options for Questions 148 – 150

A. 3-0 Polyglactin sutures	F. Vicryl rapid sutures + End to end technique
B. 3-0 Vicryl rapid sutures	G. Vicryl rapid sutures + Figure of eight suture
C. Polydioxanone (PDS) sutures + Figure of eight suture	H. 3-0 Polydioxanone (PDS) sutures + Overlap technique
D. 3-0 Polyglactin sutures + Figure of eight suture	I. 3-0 Polydioxanone (PDS) sutures + End to end technique
E. 2-0 Vicryl rapid sutures + Overlap technique	J. 2-0 Polyglactin sutures + Overlap technique

Instructions

For each case described below, choose the single most likely suturing material and technique from the above list of options. Each option may be used once, more than once, or not at all.

148) A 35 year old woman was delivered by Neville Barnes Forceps. On vaginal and rectal examination, she was found to have a tear involving the internal and external sphincter. The rectal mucosa is intact.

149) A 25 year-old multiparous woman had a normal delivery. When the midwife started suturing, she could see the tear extending to the anal mucosa. On further examination by the doctor this was confirmed.

150) A 25 year-old primiparous woman has a spontaneous vaginal delivery with a tear involving her vagina. On further examination, the external anal sphincter was partially torn.

Options for Questions 151 -156

A. Pulmonary embolism	G. Heart failure
B. Asthma	H. Anxiety
C. Physiological changes in pregnancy	I. Pulmonary oedema
D. Anaemia	J. Pneumonia
E. Polyhydramnios	K. Pneumothorax
F. Oedema	

Instructions

For the following case scenarios, please choose the single most likely cause of shortness of breath from the above list of options. Each option may be used once, more than once, or not at all.

151) A 34year old G1P0 is admitted at 25 weeks gestation with breathlessness two days after a transAtlantic flight. She has no fever and her BMI is 34kg/m2. BP 110/78mmHg, Pulse 105bpm, O_2 saturation 95%.

152) A 40 year old woman with essential hypertension is admitted with gradually increasing shortness of breath. She is 30 weeks pregnant and has bilateral pedal oedema and mild hepatomegaly. BP 130/88, Pulse 90/min, O_2 saturation 96%, RR 28/min.

153) A 28 year old G3P4, 36weeks pregnant with DCDA twins is admitted with gradually increasing shortness of breath, tiredness and headache. BP 108/66mmHG, Pulse 86bpm, O_2 saturation 98%.

154) A 29 year old G2P1 with gestational diabetes is seen in triage with increasing shortness of breath and it is difficult to palpate fetal parts. She has a BMI of 28kg/m^2. BP 110/70mmHg, Pulse 88bpm, O_2 saturation 99%.

155) A 30year old G5P4 is admitted with feeling unwell, right upper quadrant pain, breathlessness and a week's history of productive cough. T 37.8°C, BP 100/60mmHg, Pulse 109bpm. O_2 saturation 96%.

156) A 27 year old G1P0 presents with shortness of breath after having her anomaly scan which revealed cleft lip of the baby. BP 100/70mmHg, Pulse 100bpm, O_2 saturation 98%.

Options for Questions 157 -161

A. Placental abruption	G. Appendicitis
B. Chorioamnionitis	H. Ovarian cyst
C. Musculoskeletal pain	I. Gastroenteritis
D. Urinary tract infection	J. Degenerating fibroid
E. Pancreatitis	K. Gallstones
F. Adhesions	

Instructions

For the following case scenarios, please choose the single most likely cause of abdominal pain from the above list of options. Each option may be used once, more than once, or not at all.

157) A 25 year old G3P2 is admitted at 18 weeks gestation with a 5-day history of abdominal pain mainly around the umbilicus, feeling unwell and nausea. She is tender on palpating the

abdomen especially at the right lower quadrant. BP 108/60mmHg. Pulse 102bpm. Temp 38°C.

158) A 16 year G1P0 is admitted with moderate abdominal pain and vomiting. The pain is colicky in nature. BP 100/70mmHg, Pulse 92/min. T 37°C.

159) A 30 year old G1P0 is admitted with sudden onset abdominal pain and reduced fetal movement at 32 weeks gestation. BP 150/98mmHg. Pulse 100/min. T 36.8°C.

160) A 34 year old G2P1 presents with gradual onset abdominal pain of a week's duration. The pain is worse on movement. She has no nausea or vomiting and there is no tenderness on palpating the abdomen. Her dating ultrasound showed a 1.5cm left simple ovarian cyst. BP 110/70mmHg, Pulse 82/min, T 37°C.

161) A 35 year old G1P0 with a previous myomectomy is admitted with abdominal pain at 26 weeks gestation. The pain is worse on the left side. The symphysio - fundal height is 30cm and the uterus seem deviated to the left. BP 105/78mmHg. Pulse 100/min. T 37.1°C.

Options for Questions 162 -167

A Artificial rupture of membranes (ARM)	F. Catheter balloon insertion
B. Start syntocinon infusion	G. Stabilizing induction
C. Propess	H. Caesarean section
D. Prostin	I. Expectant management
E. Misoprostol	J. Membrane sweep

Instructions

For the following case scenarios, please choose the single best method of induction from the above list of options. Each option may be used once, more than once, or not at all

162) A 30 year old G1P0 with an uncomplicated pregnancy attends the antenatal clinic at 40 weeks gestation to discuss induction of labour.

163) A 31 year old G2P1 who delivered by caesarean section presents at 40 weeks and 4 days gestation to the antenatal ward for induction of labour. She has a bishop score of 5.

164) A 37 year old G5P4 with 3 vaginal deliveries followed by a caesarean section for breech presentation presents to the labour ward with spontaneous rupture of membranes 27 hours ago at 39 weeks gestation. She is not contracting and draining clear amniotic fluid. The cervix is 2cm dilated on examination.

165) A 22 year old GIPO at 37 weeks gestation has an ultrasound, which shows the abdominal circumference to be below the 3rd centile, estimated fetal weight of 1999gm and Umbilical Artery Doppler showing absent end diastolic flow. Her bishop score is 7 on vaginal examination.

166) A 30 year old G3P2 with history of uncomplicated vaginal deliveries attend the antenatal clinic at 39 weeks gestation to discuss delivery. She has history of 2 precipitate labours.

167) A 32 year old G2P1 who had a previous caesarean section for fetal distress at term presents to labour ward at 27 weeks gestation with no fetal movements. She is diagnosed to have an intrauterine fetal death.

Options for Questions 168 -173

A. Caesarean section grade 2	G. Stop syntocinon
B. Caesarean section grade 1	H. Subcutaneous terbutaline
C. Reassess in 2 hours	I. External cephalic version
D. Reassess in 4 hours	J. Repeat induction process
E. Artificial rupture of membranes	K. Membrane sweep
F. Artificial rupture of membranes and syntocinon	

Instructions

For the following case scenarios, please choose the single most appropriate next intervention from the above list of options. Each option may be used once, more than once, or not at all.

168) A 36 year old G1P0 in established labour is seen on the labour ward. She is having 4 contractions every 10 min. No liquor has been seen. Cervical dilatation was 4 cm 4 hours ago and is now 5cm.

169) A 37 year old G2P1 is transferred from the antenatal ward to labour ward. She is having induction of labour at 41 weeks + 5 days. On examination, something pulsating is felt through the membranes. The CTG is normal and the cervix is 3cm dilated. She is not contracting.

170) A 37 year old G2P1 is transferred from the antenatal ward where she is having induction of labour at 41 weeks + 5 days to the labour ward. On rupturing the membranes, there is prolapse of the umbilical cord. The CTG is normal, cervix is 3cm dilated and she is not contracting.

171) A 32 year old G7P6 with history of 6 vaginal deliveries is seen on the labour ward. She 41 + 6 weeks and having is 2 contractions every 10mins. Cervical dilatation is 6cm at present. It was 5cm with a fully effaced cervix 4 hours ago and 4 cm 8 hours ago while she was on the antenatal ward.

172) A 25 year G2P0 who is 37 weeks pregnant is having induction of labour for Obstetric Cholestasis. She had propess followed by 3 mg of prostin. The Bishops score remains 1. She has a history of multiple abdominal surgeries as a child.

173) A 32 years G1P0 comes with a history of spontaneous rupture of membranes and in labour. She is 8 cm dilated and on examination the position of the fetus is left occipito transverse. The station is -1. There is 2+ of caput and 1+ of moulding. She is contracting 4:10. 4 hours ago she was 8 cm dilated.

Options for Questions 174 -181

A. Caesarean section grade 1	G. Ventouse (non rotational)
B. Caesarean section grade 2	H. Allow pushing for a further one hour
C. Manual rotation and ventouse	I. Fetal blood sampling
D. Forceps (non rotational)	J. Manual rotation and forceps
E. Forceps (rotational)	K. Syntocinon infusion
F. Ventouse (rotational)	L. Transfer to theatre for instrumental delivery or caesarean section

Instructions

For the following case scenarios, please choose the single best next management from the above list of options. Each option may be used once, more than once, or not at all.

174) You are called to see a primiparous woman in second stage of labour. She is 39 weeks pregnant and was fully dilated 1 hour ago. She is having irregular contractions every 4 minutes. The CTG is satisfactory. Vaginal examination shows the vertex to be in left occipito posterior position, at the level of the ischial spines. There is no caput or moulding.

175) A 30 year old woman in her second pregnancy at 40 weeks gestation has progressed well in labour and has been effectively pushing for the last 90 mins. She was fully dilated 2 and half hours ago. There is no palpable head on abdominal examination. Vaginal examination shows the vertex to be in occipito anterior position and at 2cm below the ischial spines. There is 3 + of caput and no moulding. The CTG is showing late decelerations. Her first baby was delivered by spontaneous vaginal delivery.

176) A 42 year old G1P0 is seen on the labour ward rounds. Labour has progressed well and she has been fully dilated for 2 hours and pushing for the last 1 hour. There is no palpable head on abdominal examination. Vaginal examination shows the vertex to be in left occipito anterior position and at 1cm below the ischial spines. There is 1 + of caput and no moulding. The CTG is normal. She conceived by IVF after trying for 6 yrs.

177) You are called to see a 22 year old G2P1 who has not delivered after 1 hour of effective pushing. On vaginal examination, the fetal mouth, nose and the orbital ridges can easily be felt. The chin of the foetus can also be felt and it is pointing towards the symphysis pubis of the mother. The presenting part is about 2 cm below the ischial spines. The CTG is satisfactory.

178) A 24 year old G3P2 with one previous caesarean section followed by a successful vaginal birth is seen on the labour ward at second stage of labour. She is 41 weeks pregnant and her labour has progressed well in the first stage up to 8cm. Subsequently it took her 5 hours to progress from 8cm to full dilatation. She has been pushing effectively for1 hour. On examination there is a fifth of

the fetal head palpable abdominally. On vaginal examination the vertex is in occipito transverse position with 2 + of caput and reducible moulding. The vertex is at the level of the ischial spines and the CTG is satisfactory.

179) A 34 year old G2P1 is in the 2nd stage of labour. She is 33+4 weeks gestation. On examination, the vertex is at +1 and Left occipito transverse position. CTG is abnormal.

180) You are called to see a 31 year old G2P1 with previous baby delivered by spontaneous vaginal delivery with no complications. You are asked to see her because of CTG abnormalities. The CTG shows baseline rate 170bpm, reduced variability for the last 30min and short lasting early decelerations. On vaginal examination, the cervix is found to be 10 cm dilated. It was 6 cm 2 hours ago. The vertex is at the level of the ischial spine, in occipito anterior position and there is 1+ caput and no moulding. The liquor is significantly meconium stained.

181) A 28 year old G2P1 is in spontaneous labour at 41 weeks gestation. She is having 4 contractions every 10 min and on examination the cervix is fully dilated and vertex is at +1 and occipito anterior position. She had spontaneous rupture of membrane while doing the vaginal examination and cord is felt.

Options for Questions 182 -187

A. Puerperal psychosis	G. Breast abscess
B. Meningitis	H. Pyelonephritis
C. Post-natal blues	I. Bipolar disorder
D. Endometritis	J. Post-traumatic stress disorder
E. Sepsis	K. Post-natal depression
F. Mastitis	L. Anxiety

Instructions

For the following case scenarios, please choose the single most likely diagnosis from the above list of options. Each option may be used once, more than once, or not at all.

182) A 20 year old woman delivered 4 days ago and presents to her midwife being very tearful and anxious. She is coping well with her day to day activities, although appears quite irritable. Her temperature and vital signs are normal.

183) A 32 year old woman was brought to hospital in spontaneous labour. She developed pyrexia in labour and was delivered by caesarean section. She presented four days following the caesarean section feeling unwell. On examination her blood pressure is 110/62mmHg, pulsc is 90bpm, temperature 37.6°C. She is tender in the lower abdomen and the caesarean section wound looks healthy. She declines having a speculum or internal examination due to pain.

184) You are called to see a 40 year old schoolteacher on the postnatal ward, who has suddenly become confused and agitated three days after spontaneous vaginal delivery of her first child. The midwives tell you that she has been sleeping poorly and felt low in mood. She claims that she works at the House of Commons and will report all the staff on the ward who is trying to assault her to the police.

185) A 28 year old woman presents five days after spontaneous vaginal delivery of her second child. She presented with flu-like symptoms for the last two days, and reports a painful, swollen right breast. On examination her temperature is 38°C, pulse and blood pressure are within normal range. There is redness and engorgement of the right breast, with tenderness on palpation.

186) A 19 year old woman presents to Accident and Emergency generally feeling unwell for the past three days with malaise and rigors. She had ventouse delivery one week ago. Her blood pressure is 85/58mmHg, pulse 120bpm, and temperature is 39°C. The lochia is not offensive.

187) A 20 year old single mother is referred by her community midwife four weeks after delivery due to low mood and increasing inability to cope at home. She is not enjoying looking after her newborn child. She was treated by her GP during the antenatal period for anxiety.

Options for Questions 188 -193

A. Atopic eruption of pregnancy	G. Hyperpigmentation
B. Impetigo herpertiformis	H. Straie gravidarum
C. Intrahepatic cholestasis of pregnancy	I. Pemphigoid gestationalis
D. Prurigo of pregnancy	J. Pruritic folliculitis of pregnancy
E. Polymorphic eruption of pregnancy	K. Rubella
F. Chicken pox	

Instructions

For the following case scenarios, please choose the single most likely diagnosis from the above list of options. Each option may be used once, more than once, or not at all.

188) A 22 year old in her first pregnancy presents at 22 weeks with linear purplish marks mainly on the abdomen, thighs and buttocks. This is non itchy.

189) A 32 year old Indian lady at 33 weeks gestation complains of difficulty sleeping at night due to generalized intense itching and involving the hands, feet and abdomen. There are excoriation marks on the itchy areas and hyperpigmentation at the back due to scratching. There are no visible rashes.

190) A 30 year old G3P2 with DCDA twins at 34 weeks presents with erythematous maculopapular rash on her abdomen of 4 days duration, which has gradually spread, to the trunk. The lesions are itchy and do not affect the periumbilical area. The palms are also not affected.

191) A 40 year old woman in her second pregnancy presents at 30 weeks with blisters on the thighs. It started as a rash around the umbilicus with papules and plaques, which later forms bullous lesions spread to the other parts of the trunk and the limbs. She also suffers from hyperthyroidism.

192) A 20 year old G1P0 presents with papular and nodular rash on the face, neck and chest at 14 weeks gestation. The papules are erythematous and some of them looked excoriated. Her mother suffers from hay fever.

193) A 21year old G1P0 is seen in triage with an intensely itchy rash all over the body at 19 weeks gestation. The rash started as small erythematous papules and later develops into vesicles with fever. The rash started from the trunk spreading to the limbs. Some of the vesicles are beginning to crust over including the ones on the scalp.

Options for Questions 194 –201

A. Low molecular weight heparin (LMWH) for six weeks	G. LMWH after four hours
B. LMWH for ten days	H. LMWH after six hours
C. LMWH for seven days	I. Warfarin
D. LMWH for six months	J. Advice on mobilization and avoidance of dehydration
E. Aspirin for six weeks	K. Compression stockings
F. LMWH after two hours	L. Discuss with haematologist

Instructions

For the following case scenarios, please choose the single most appropriate management from the above list of options. Each option may be used once, more than once, or not at all.

194) A 26 year old woman with a BMI of 29 kg/m^2 has had a spontaneous vaginal delivery of her second baby. She has no medical conditions and the estimated blood loss was 500mls. She had deep vein thrombosis 5 years ago after a holiday in Singapore.

195) A 30 year old woman with a BMI of 24 kg/m^2 is about to be discharged home after delivery of her first child. She had an uncomplicated vaginal delivery with the baby weighing 4.5kg. She has gross varicosities on both legs.

196) A 28 year old woman with a mechanical heart valve is being discharged from hospital after the delivery of her third baby by forceps. The estimated blood loss was 1100mls. She delivered 8 days ago and had stayed in hospital as her baby was in the

neonatal unit. She is on anticoagulation. She wants to continue breastfeeding her baby.

197) A healthy 28 year old woman has had an elective caesarean section for a breech presentation and is about to go home two days after the surgery. The caesarean section was uncomplicated and the estimated blood loss was 500mls. Her BMI is 29.5kg/m^2.

198) A 31 year old woman had a normal vaginal delivery of a male infant four days ago. She has been readmitted to hospital with mastitis for which she had antibiotic and about to be discharged 4 days after admission. This was her first pregnancy and her BMI is 27kg/m^2.

199) A 25 year woman G2P1 attended the maternity unit with no fetal movements for 24 hours. She had a spontaneous vaginal delivery of a macerated baby after rupturing her membranes and going into spontaneous labour. She has a BMI of 28kg/m^2 and smokes 8 cigarettes a day. She is about to be discharged home from the labour ward.

200) A 21 year dancer has had a preterm delivery after spontaneously rupturing her membranes at 33 weeks. She went into spontaneous labour whiles being managed conservatively. Her BMI is 21 kg/m^2 and this was her fourth pregnancy after having three previous miscarriages. As part of the investigations for the miscarriage she was found to have Antithrombin deficiency. There is no past or present medical condition of note.

201) A 42 year old woman with a BMI of 35kg/m^2 has just had a caesarean section to deliver her third baby due to fetal distress. She had epidural for analgesia during labour. The caesarean section was uncomplicated and the estimated blood loss was 600mls. The epidural catheter has just been removed and she is due to have LMWH.

Chapter 4

SINGLE BEST ANSWERS (SBAS)

1. A 27 year old lady has undergone a transcervical resection of fibroid for a 4 cm fibroid. She is undergoing fertility investigations.

Which of the following anti adhesive agents should be used to prevent intrauterine adhesions?

A. Hydrocortisone infusion
B. Prednisolone infusion
C. Heparin
D. Hyaluronan gel
E. Icodextrin

2. An 83 year old lady is admitted with abdominal distention and pain. She is found to have gross ascites with an ovarian mass.

Which of the following is the physiological process responsible for her ascites?

A. Compression of hepatic vein
B. Increased permeability of capillaries
C. Decreased production of fluid
D. Increased lymphatic flow to 100mls/hr.
E. Compression of portal vein

3. A woman with a BMI of 55 is planning for bariatric surgery. Which of the following is a malabsorptive procedure?

A. Laparoscopic adjustable gastric banding
B. Silastic ring gastroplasty
C. Roux-en-Y gastric bypass
D. Vertical banded gastroplasty
E. Sleeve gastrectomy

4. There is good evidence that bariatric surgery improves the following in women except:

A. Miscarriage rate
B. Success rate of IVF
C. Resolution of PCOS rate
D. Maternal outcome
E. Fetal outcome

5. A 60 year old woman is experiencing post menopausal bleeding. Her BMI is 45.

Which of the following type of cancer is she at risk of?

A. Carcinosarcoma
B. Serous endometrial cancer
C. Endometrioid endometrial cancer
D. Clear cell carcinoma
E. Adenocarcinoma

6. A 65 year old woman with a BMI of 42 presents with postmenopausal bleeding. On pipelle biopsy she is found to have endometrioid endometrial cancer. The MRI scan confirms the malignancy to be confined to the one half of the myometrium.

What is the first line of management for her?

A. Brachytherapy
B. Total abdominal hysterectomy + Bilateral salpingo-oophorectomy
C. Laparoscopic hysterectomy + Bilateral salpingo-oophorectomy

D. Mirena IUS
E. Chemotherapy

7. A 56 year old woman undergoes total abdominal hysterectomy for fibroid uterus.

Following is one of the steps for her enhanced recovery:

A. Clear fluid up to 4 hours prior to surgery
B. Long acting sedative premedication
C. Administration of antibiotic after the completion of surgery
D. Thromboprophylaxis
E. Increase the volume of intravenous fluid

8. A 26 year old woman is diagnosed with cervical cancer.

How many women in UK are diagnosed with cervical cancer annually before the age of 45?

A. 1500
B. 1000
C. 500
D. 100
E. 2000

9. A 26 year old diagnosed with squamous cell cancer of the cervix. She is nulliparous. She has a 2cm tumour on her cervix.

What should be the appropriate management?

A. Radical vaginal trachelectomy
B. Radical abdominal trachelectomy
C. Neoadjuvant chemotherapy + Cone biopsy
D. Ovarian transposition and radiotherapy
E. Cone biopsy

10. A 34 year old is diagnosed CIN3 on colposcopy and CIN2 on cervical punch biopsy. She is adamant that she wants an ablation technique rather than an excision.

Following is the reason, why she will not be suitable for an ablation method.

A. Her entire transformation zone is not visible
B. The colposcopic and histology diagnosis are different
C. There is no evidence for glandular disease
D. There is no evidence of invasive disease
E. Her age is lower than 50

11. A 53 year old postmenopausal woman has CIN2 on colposcopy and cervical biopsy. She has a type 3 transformation zone and is due to have LLETZ procedure.

Following is the depth/length of the tissue that should be removed.

A. 5 – 10 mm
B. 10 – 15mm
C. 20 - 30mm
D. 15 – 20 mm
E. 15- 25mm

12. A 27 year old is diagnosed with CIN1 and is on regular colposcopic monitoring. She is now 13 weeks pregnant.

What should be her management?

A. Colposcopy should deferred till delivery
B. Colposcopy should be performed now
C. Colposcopy at 3rd trimester
D. Cervical smear now
E. HPV testing can be performed

13. A 41 year old lady has been diagnosed with estrogen positive breast cancer. She is 16 weeks pregnant at present.

What should be the management?

A. Breast conserving surgery should not be undertaken until 28 weeks
B. Systemic Chemotherapy can be given to this patient

C. Tamoxifen can be used after surgery
D. Axillary lymph node clearance should be deferred till delivery if axilla is positive
E. Radiotherapy can be given after 28 weeks if indicated

14. A 38 year old lady has been diagnosed with ER negative breast cancer. She received adjuvant chemotherapy. She is planning to conceive her 2nd child.

What should be the plan for further management?

A. She should wait for at least 5 years
B. She should be counselled that there is a slightly increased risk of congenital anomalies in the fetus
C. ECHO should be performed in pregnancy to detect cardiomyopathy
D. She should be advised to avoid breastfeeding.
E. She can be assured that fertility is not affected following breast cancer treatment.

15. A 46 year old woman complains of menorrhagia. She is diagnosed to have endometrial hyperplasia without atypia.

The risk of her disease progressing to endometrial cancer is:

A. 5% over 10 years
B. <5% over 15 years
C. <5% over 20 years
D. 5% over 5 years
E. 5% over 20 years

16. A 50 year old woman complains of menorrhagia.

The gold standard investigation for her is:

A. Transvaginal Ultrasound Scan
B. Diffusion weighted Magnetic Resonance Imaging
C. Computed Tomography
D. Endometrial Pipelle Biopsy
E. Hysteroscopy & Endometrial Biopsy

17. A 59 year old para 2 woman presented with postmenopausal bleeding. She was found to have an endometrial thickness of 11mm on ultrasound scan. She was booked for an outpatient hysteroscopy.

What size of hysteroscope should be used for her procedure?

A. 3mm hysteroscope with 4.5 - 5mm sheath
B. 3.3mm hysteroscope with 4.5 - 5mm sheath
C. 3.0mm hysteroscope with 4 - 5mm sheath
D. 2.5mm hysteroscope with 3.5 - 4mm sheath
E. 2.7mm hysteroscope with 3 – 3.5mm sheath

18. A 49 year old woman is undergoing outpatient hysteroscopy and polyp resection using electrosurgery.

Please choose the best distention medium that will reduce her risk of having vasovagal attack.

A. Normal Saline
B. Glycine
C. CO2
D. Mannitol
E. Glucose

19. A 34 year old woman was admitted for a diagnostic laparoscopy for investigation for subfertility. She weighed 65kg and was fit and healthy. The Senior House Officer was performing the procedure under direct supervision by the Consultant.

What should be the angle at which the primary trocar is inserted?

A. 15° towards the pelvis
B. 30° towards the pelvis
C. 45° to the skin
D. 60° to the skin
E. 90° to the skin

20. A 28 year old woman has been admitted in emergency with ectopic pregnancy and needs laparoscopic salpingectomy. She gives history of previous midline laparotomy for bowel surgery.

What would be the best method for verress needle insertion?

A. Direct trocar entry
B. Palmer's point entry
C. Suprapubic entry
D. Posterior fornix entry
E. Entry with visual access system

21. A 21 year old young woman is booked for diagnostic laparoscopy for chronic pelvic pain. Her BMI is 19.

Her highest risk of complication is:

A. Intestinal Injury
B. Splenic injury
C. Bladder injury
D. Vascular injury
E. Hernia formation

22. A woman is booked in for marsupialization of bartholin's cyst. She is being brought into theatre after having an anesthetic.

The following should be checked as per the WHO surgical checklist

A. Blood group of the patient
B. Urine pregnancy test
C. Patient specific concern
D. Need for catheter
E. Patient positioning

23. A woman is booked in for marsupialization of bartholin's cyst. She is being brought into theatre.

Which of the following should be checked prior to induction on anesthesia as per the WHO surgical checklist?

A. Allergy status
B. Equipment sterility
C. Antibiotic requirement
D. Glycemic control
E. ASA Grade

24. Mrs. Smith is 46 and has been diagnosed with an ovarian cyst that causes her pain. Her risk of the cyst being malignant at present is 1:1000.

What would be the risk of malignancy when she turns 50?

A. 2:1000
B. 1:1000
C. 3:1000
D. 4:1000
E. 5:1000

25. A 34 year old lady presents with generalized abdominal pain after laparoscopic ovarian cystectomy for 12 cm dermoid cyst. There was considerable amount of spillage of contents during surgery. The biochemistry shows raised CRP and a diagnosis of chemical peritonitis is made.

The incidence of chemical peritonitis is:

A. 0.1%
B. 0.5%
C. 0.2%
D. 0.25%
E. 0.75%

26. A 39 year old para 3 lady wants female sterilization. She is being consented prior to surgery.

What would be the failure risk of hysteroscopic sterilization?

A. 1 in 10000
B. 1 in 1000

C. 2 in 10000
D. 2 in 1000
E. 2 in 100

27. A 65 year old lady is diagnosed with epithelial ovarian cancer confined to the fallopian tube and ovary.

Her 5-year survival rate is:

A. 70- 75%
B. 80 – 85%
C. 85 – 90%
D. 80- 95%
E. 80 – 90%

28. A 64 year old woman is suspected to have Stage 1 ovarian cancer.

She should have the following as first line management.

A. Adjuvant chemotherapy
B. Staging surgery with Retroperitoneal lymph node assessment
C. Staging surgery with Systemic retroperitoneal lymphadenectomy
D. Staging surgery
E. Radiotherapy

29. A staging laparotomy for ovarian cancer involves the following:

A. Laparotomy + Total abdominal hysterectomy (TAH) + Bilateral salpingo-oophorectomy (BSO) + Biopsies of peritoneal deposit + Biopsy of pelvic & abdominal peritoneum + retroperitoneal lymph node assessment
B. Laparotomy + TAH + BSO + Infracolic Omentectomy + Biopsy of pelvic & abdominal peritoneum + retroperitoneal lymph node assessment
C. Laparotomy + TAH + BSO + Infracolic Omentectomy + Biopsies of peritoneal deposit + Biopsy of abdominal peritoneum + retroperitoneal lymph node assessment

D. Laparotomy + TAH + BSO + Infracolic Omentectomy + Biopsies of peritoneal deposit + Biopsy of pelvic peritoneum + retroperitoneal lymph node assessment
E. Laparotomy + TAH + BSO + Infracolic Omentectomy + Biopsies of peritoneal deposit + Biopsy of pelvic & abdominal peritoneum + retroperitoneal lymph node assessment

30. A 59 year old lady is diagnosed with high risk Stage 1c Ovarian cancer (Grade 3)

She is offered adjuvant chemotherapy with:

A. 5 cycles of carboplatin
B. 5 cycles of paclitaxel
C. 6 cycles of carboplatin
D. 6 cycles of paclitaxel
E. 6 cycles of cisplatin

31. A 49 year old woman has total abdominal hysterectomy for endometrial cancer. The histology confirms that the tumour invades the serosa.

The FIGO staging is:

A. Stage II
B. Stage IIIA
C. Stage IIIB
D. Stage IIIC1
E. Stage IIIC2

32. A 70 year old is diagnosed with vulval cancer. She gives history of lichen sclerosis.

What percentage of vulval cancer has association with lichen sclerosis?

A. 30%
B. 31%
C. 32%

D. 33%
E. 34%

33. A 70 year old is diagnosed with vulval cancer. She had wide local excision and lymphadenectomy for staging.

The following lymph node excision has the lowest morbidity:

A. Radical lymphadenectomy
B. Sentinel node biopsy
C. Systemic inguino femoral node dissection
D. Femoral node dissection
E. Para aortic node dissection

34. A 64 year old lady is having ovarian debulking surgery.

The disadvantages of her having a midline incision is as follows:

A. Median incision is more hemorrhagic
B. There is major nerve damages
C. The abdomen and pelvis can be entered rapidly
D. Wound dehiscence risk is higher
E. She will have better cosmetic result

35. A 26 year old lady is having cervical suture with Mersilene tape.

The following is a characteristic of the Mersilene tape:

A. It has high tissue reaction
B. It is a monofilament suture
C. It has a high tensile strength
D. The handling of the material is difficult
E. It gets absorbed in 150 days

36. Mrs. Page needs a suprapubic catheter for neurogenic bladder.

Which of the following material should the suprapubic catheter be made of to reduce complications?

A. Latex
B. Siliconised latex
C. Plastic/PVC
D. Latex coated with Teflon
E. 100% silicone

37. A 67 year old lady is having suprapubic catheterization following a gynaecological surgery.

Following is a contraindication for the same:

A. Neurogenic Bladder
B. Inability to mobilize
C. Urethral stricture
D. Chronic retention
E. Anticoagulation therapy for blood clotting disorder

38. A 52 year old woman had laparoscopic assisted vaginal hysterectomy. She sustained a bladder injury during the procedure that was repaired laparoscopically. The approximate incidence of fistula formation is:

A. 5%
B. 5.5%
C. 6%
D. 6.5%
E. 7%

39. A 65 year old lady had a major transection ureteric injury during abdominal hysterectomy for large fibroid uterus. The injury in the upper 1/3rd of the ureter.

The following method should be used for repair:

A. Uretero-ureterostomy
B. Trans - Uretero-ureterostomy
C. uretero-neocystostomy
D. Psoas hitch
E. Boari Flap

40. A 54 year old sustained bladder injury during laparoscopic assisted vaginal hysterectomy. She had the catheter for 2 weeks. Prior to removal of the catheter she needs:

A. Cystoscopy
B. Micturating cystourethrogram
C. MRI
D. CT Scan Pelvis
E. Retrograde cystography

41. A 65 year old lady is having debulking surgery for ovarian cancer. Excision of external iliac nodes was carried out. 2 months later, she presented with paraesthesia over mons pubis and labia.

Which nerve injury did she sustain during the surgery?

A. Iliohypogastric Nerve
B. Obturator Nerve
C. Genitofemoral Nerve
D. Lateral Cutaneous Nerve
E. Pudendal Nerve

42. A 70 year old lady is undergoing hysteroscopy with a 30° hysteroscope. She has a retroverted uterus. What should be the position of the cervical os on view for appropriate hydrodilatation?

A. 6 o'clock with the light cable up
B. 9 o'clock with the light cable down
C. 12 o'clock with the light cable up
D. 12 o'clock with the light cable down
E. Central

43. A 43 year old 6 weeks pregnant lady is admitted to A&E Resuscitation area with hypotension, tachycardia and severe abdominal pain. A diagnosis of ruptured ectopic pregnancy is made and the decision for laparoscopy +/- salpingectomy is made. After discussion with her mother, she refuses to consent for the procedure.

The Court of Protection could be approached as:

A. She lacks capacity as she refuses surgery even though she is critical
B. She lacks capacity as she is in severe pain
C. Her refusal is not valid as she is influenced by her mother
D. She lacks capacity as she is haemodynamically unstable
E. Her refusal is not valid as she is pregnant.

44. A 44 year old lady with BMI of 40 kg/m2 has a total abdominal hysterectomy. The procedure was complex as the uterus was 18 weeks size due to multiple fibroids. She presents with chest pain and hemoptysis 4 days later.

The following ECG changes may suggest pulmonary embolism:

A. S wave in lead 1; Q wave in lead 3, Inverted T wave in lead 3
B. S wave in lead 3, Q wave in lead 3, T wave in lead 1
C. S wave in lead 1, Q wave in lead 1, Inverted T wave in lead 3
D. S wave in lead 2, Q wave in lead 1, Inverted T wave in lead 3
E. S wave in lead 1, Q wave in lead 2, Inverted T wave in lead 1

45. A 28 year old lady presents with a pelvic mass. She also complains of hirsutism and voice change. Her testosterone level is 9nmol/L.

She is suspected to have the following type of ovarian tumor:

A. Granulosa cell tumor
B. Leydig cell tumor
C. Clear cell tumour
D. Endometrioid ovarian cancer
E. Borderline tumor

46. A ST7 trainee is reviewing the risk reporting system in gynaecology.

Following incident need not be included in the trigger list:

A. Delayed diagnosis of ectopic pregnancy
B. Pneumothorax during laparoscopy
C. Unplanned admission to ITU

D. Blood loss of 400mls during hysterectomy
E. Conflict between surgeons regarding management of case

47. Every trust should have a risk management team for a particular specialty.

The following personnel should be part of a gynaecology risk team except:

A. Consultant Gynaecologist
B. Ultrasonographer
C. Theatre Practitioner
D. Service Manager
E. MDT Coordinator

48. A ST4 trainee is performing an audit on the outcome of Group B streptococcus infection in Obstetric patients.

She should be proceeding in the following sequence:

A. Identify a standard, Collect data to assess performance, Implement the changes if there is any, Collect data to determine whether care has been improved
B. Collect data to assess performance, Identify a standard, Implement the changes if there is any, Collect data to determine whether care has been improved
C. Collect data to assess performance, Identify a standard, Collect data to determine whether care has been improved, Implement the changes if there is any
D. Identify a standard, Implement the changes if there is any, Collect data to assess performance, Collect data to determine whether care has been improved
E. Collect data to determine whether care has been improved, Collect data to assess performance, Identify a standard, Implement the changes if there is any

49. An audit is being done where the methods of induction of labour are being compared.

The statistical test to compare two sets of observations on a single sample would be:

A. Mann-Whitney U test
B. Wilcoxon matched pairs test
C. Kruskall-Wallis analysis of variance by ranks
D. Fishers's exact test
E. Spearman's rank correlation coefficient (rσ)

50. A study is designed to compare the age distribution in patients presenting with ectopic pregnancy. The null hypothesis is that there is no difference in the age groups of women presenting with ectopic pregnancy.

The appropriate statistical test is:

A. Two sample unpaired t-test
B. One sample paired t-test
C. X_2 test
D. Pearson's r test
E. F test

51. A researcher wants to measure the incidence of angular pregnancy. The following research methodology should be used:

A. Case control study
B. Cohort study
C. Randomised controlled study
D. Cross sectional descriptive study
E. Longitudinal descriptive study

52. A researcher wants to obtain evidence of association of exposure of pregnant women to passive smoking and the outcome.

The following research method is appropriate:

A. Case control study
B. Cohort study
C. Randomised controlled study

D. Cross sectional descriptive study
E. Longitudinal descriptive study

53. A 34 year old lady presents to with secondary subfertility. She has been trying to conceive for 6 months and gives history of regular normal periods. On investigations, her FSH is 16 IU/L, LH is 10IU/L and AMH is 3ng/ml. Antral follicle count is 3.

Choose a single option that best suits her treatment option.

A. Await 6 months prior to referral to fertility clinic
B. Clomiphene ovulation induction
C. IVF
D. Gonadotrophin stimulation & IUI
E. Donor Egg IVF

54. A 32 year old woman with a BMI of 34 and oligomenorrhoea is diagnosed to have polycystic ovarian syndrome. Regarding her risk factors for developing cancer.

The following statement is true:

A. Endometrial thickness greater than 7 mm may be hyperplasia
B. It is important to induce withdrawal bleed every 6 month
C. There is association with breast cancer
D. There is association with ovarian cancer
E. If endometrium is thickened, progesterone therapy should be instituted

55. A 28 year old woman present to the fertility clinic in secondary care with a history of oligomenorrhoea. Her BMI is 30 kg/m2. She is trying for 3 years. Her hormonal profile is normal. Tubes are patent bilaterally and husband's semen analysis is normal. She has tried clomiphene for 6 cycles but with no response (anovulatory).

The next treatment option is:

A. Metformin
B. Further 6 cycles of clomiphene at increasing dose or changing to tamoxifen
C. Ovarian Drilling
D. IVF
E. IUI

56. A 33 year old woman who is a CEO of a multinational company presents with oligomenorrhoea for 6 months. She is fit and healthy with a BMI of 24 kg/m2. Her tubal patency test and partner's semen analysis are normal. Her FSH is 2 IU/L, LH is 2 IU/L and Oestradiol is 500 IU/L.

The single best treatment option is:

A. Clomiphene
B. Metformin
C. Gonadotrophin
D. IUI
E. IVF

57. A 32 year old woman with a BMI of 29 kg/m2, presented with secondary subfertility. She has 2 children. She had a 3rd degree tear during her first childbirth and a massive obstetric haemorrhage of 5 litres during her second delivery. She is trying to conceive for 2 years. She has been amenorrhoic since her last childbirth.

The best option is:

A. Clomiphene
B. IVF
C. Gonadotrophin
D. Donor egg
E. Pulsatile GnRH

58. A 32 year old nulliparous lady trying to conceive for 3 years. All routine investigations on her and her partner reveal no abnormality.

What should be the next line of management?

A. Clomiphene ovulation induction
B. IUI
C. IUI with clomiphene induction of ovulation
D. IUI with gonadotrophin induction of ovulation
E. IVF

59. A 30 year old woman has been trying to conceive for 2 years. Her partner's semen analysis is normal as is her hormonal profile, tubal patency test and pelvic ultrasound. Her luteal phase progesterone is ovulatory. She had deep dyspareunia and mild dysmenorrhoea and had a laparoscopy where peritoneal endometriosis was ablated 6 months ago. ASA Stage 1 endometriosis was diagnosed.

What should be the next line of management?

A. Clomiphene ovulation induction
B. IUI
C. IUI with clomiphene induction of ovulation
D. IUI with gonadotrophin induction of ovulation
E. IVF

60. A 28 year old woman has irregular, heavy periods. For the last 6 months, she bleeds every 14 days for 7 days. She presented with secondary subfertility.

The endocrine/blood test necessary is:

A. Prolactin
B. FSH
C. Testosterone
D. Thyroid Function Test
E. Day 21 progesterone

61. A 26 year old woman presented with primary subfertility. Her hormonal profile is normal and luteal phase progesterone is ovulatory. Her pelvic ultrasound scan suggests a subseptate uterus but is otherwise normal. She is anxious and wants to discuss her tubal patency test.

The best option for her is:

A. 3D ultrasound scan
B. Hysteroscopy, Laparoscopy & Dye test
C. Laparoscopy & Dye test
D. Hysterosalpingogram
E. Hydrosonogram

62. A 24 year old woman had methotrexate for left tubal ectopic pregnancy. She says her G.P. has treated her once for suspected PID but the swabs were negative in GUM clinic.

Best Investigation for tubal patency is:

A. 2D & 3D ultrasound scan
B. Hysteroscopy, Laparoscopy & Dye test
C. Laparoscopy & Dye test
D. Hysterosalpingogram
E. Hydrosonogram

63. A 25 year old man presenting with gross oligozoospermia in fertility clinic. His FSH, LH, Testosterone are low. He had delayed puberty.

What is the most appropriate treatment?

A. Gonadotrophin
B. Bromocriptine/Cabergoline
C. Androgen
D. Steroids
E. IVF/ICSI

64. A 32 year old man had decreased sperm motility and count on 2 occasions and undergone semen analysis abroad. The Anti sperm antibodies are high.

What is the appropriate management?

A. Gonadotrophin
B. Bromocriptine/Cabergoline

C. Androgen
D. Steroids
E. IVF/ICSI

65. A 28 year old woman is undergoing IVF for unexplained subfertility of 3 years duration.

During treatment cycle, the following treatment is recommended well into late first trimester of pregnancy:

A. Low dose aspirin
B. Heparin
C. HCG
D. Progesterone
E. Steroids

66. A 28 year old woman and her 30 year old partner are being investigated for primary subfertility. Investigations show anovulation as the only problem. She has WHO Group 1 ovulatory disorders.

Gonadotrophin therapy should include:

A. Low dose aspirin
B. Heparin
C. HCG
D. Progesterone
E. Steroids

67. A 28 year old is being counselled after diagnosis of left tubal ectopic pregnancy.

The rate of ectopic pregnancy in U.K. is:

A. 9/1000 pregnancies
B. 10/1000 pregnancies
C. 11/1000 pregnancies
D. 12/1000 pregnancies
E. 13/1000 pregnancies

68. Maternal mortality rate due to ectopic pregnancy in U.K. is:

A. 0.5/1000 estimated ectopic pregnancies
B. 0.1/1000 estimated ectopic pregnancies
C. 0.2/1000 estimated ectopic pregnancies
D. 0.3/1000 estimated ectopic pregnancies
E. 0.4/1000 estimated ectopic pregnancies

69. A 25-year-old woman presents to early pregnancy assessment unit with minimal vaginal spotting in her first pregnancy. She is medically fit and healthy. Transvaginal ultrasound confirms a missed miscarriage of 7 weeks gestation. Clinical observations are normal.

The most appropriate immediate management option is:

A. Surgical evacuation under GA that day
B. Surgical evacuation under G.A. Next available list
C. Vacuum aspiration under Local anaesthesia
D. Medical management
E. Expectant management

70. A 25-year-old woman with no significant medical history presents at 4 + 6 weeks gestation in her first pregnancy with mild vaginal bleeding. She does not have abdominal pain.

She should be offered:

A. Transvaginal ultrasound that day
B. Transvaginal ultrasound: earliest feasible
C. Repeat urine pregnancy test in 1 week
D. Review in early pregnancy unit within 24 hours
E. Serum HCG follow up

71. A woman presents to EPAU at 7 weeks gestation with mild vaginal bleeding and abdominal cramps. She declines transvaginal scan. A transabdominal ultrasound scan shows an intrauterine gestation sac with yolk sac and foetal pole. Crown rump length is 7 mm. No foetal heart activity is seen.

She should be offered:

A. Surgical management of miscarriage
B. Medical management of miscarriage
C. Expectant management of miscarriage
D. Repeat ultrasound in 1 week
E. Repeat ultrasound in 2 weeks

72. A 28-year-old woman presents with vaginal spotting but no abdominal pain. A transvaginal ultrasound scan gives a diagnosis of Pregnancy of unknown location. 3 Serum HCG levels at 48 hours intervals are: 386, 350, and 302 mIU/ml.

The best option is:

A. Add serum progesterone
B. Repeat HCG in 48 hours
C. Repeat HCG (urine or serum) in 1 week
D. Repeat Transvaginal scan
E. Review by Senior gynaecologist

73. A 32-year-old woman presents with mild vaginal bleeding and abdominal cramps in her second pregnancy. She has a transvaginal scan and found to have a miscarriage corresponding to 8 weeks gestation. She prefers medical management.

The best option is:

A. Mifepristone 200 mg oral, followed 6 hours later by Misoprostol 800 mcg vaginal
B. Mifepristone 200 mg oral followed 24 – 36 hours later by Misoprostol 800 mcg vaginal
C. Misoprostol 400 mcg vaginal
D. Misoprostol 800 mcg oral
E. Methotrexate 600 mcg vaginal

74. A 17-year-old young woman has a transvaginal ultrasound and the diagnosis of a left tubal ectopic pregnancy is made. She does not want surgery and understands risks and agrees to follow up.

She can have methotrexate if:

A. Lower abdominal pain needing analgesia; HCG <1500 IU/ml, mass 30 mm
B. Mild lower abdominal discomfort; HCG 4500 IU/ml and left adnexal mass 32 mm
C. No pain; HCG 2000 IU/ml and left adnexal mass 36 mm
D. No pain, HCG < 1500IU/ml, mass 15 mm, echogenic free fluid in the pouch of douglas
E. No pain; HCG 5000 IU/ml; mass: 15 mm

75. A 25-year-old woman with a previous left salpingectomy for ectopic pregnancy is undergoing laparoscopy for a right tubal ectopic pregnancy. She prefers salpingotomy. She should be made aware of the possibility of further treatment in the form of methotrexate or laparoscopy.

The risks of needing further treatment is:

A. 1:2
B. 1:3
C. 1:4
D. 1:5
E. 1:6

76. A 33 year old IT professional has a job that involves sitting infront of a computer monitor for long hours and presents with 3 consecutive 1st trimester miscarriages. She drinks 10 cups of coffee and smokes 10 cigarettes a day. All her 3 previous conceptions were with her husband who is a 48 year old IT professional.

The most likely risk factor is:

A. Her occupation
B. Her age
C. Her husband's age
D. Smoking
E. Caffeine

77. In women with recurrent miscarriage, antiphospholipid antibodies are present in:

A. 2%
B. 5%
C. 10%
D. 15%
E. 25%

78. A 26-year-old woman presents to the early pregnancy unit with a third consecutive 1st trimester miscarriage. Along with the products of conception being sent for histology, a chromosomal analysis is also being requested. She has already been referred to the recurrent miscarriage clinic. She wants the investigations to be ordered now, to avoid delay.

The following investigation is necessary:

A. Factor V Leiden
B. Protein S deficiency
C. Parental karyotype
D. Lupus anticoagulant
E. 3D ultrasound

79. Mrs. Green's urodynamic results are as follows. She has initial residual volume of 90 ml and 1st desire to void at 140 ml. Her maximum capacity is 380 ml. During filling phase, systolic detrusor activity is seen which increased with tap water but not with cough in supine position. She did leak a little urine during repeated coughing in the erect posture. She had a Keilland forceps delivery 10 years ago and since then has urinary leakage on standing and straining mostly. She also wakes up at night a few times to go to the toilet.

What is the likely diagnosis?

A. Genuine stress incontinence
B. Detrusor overactivity
C. Painful bladder syndrome/ sensory urgency

D. Interstitial cystitis
E. Atonic Bladder

80. A 35 year old women presents with a history of frequency, urgency, nocturia and occasional suprapubic pain. Urodynamic investigations shows: 1st urge to void at 100 ml. There was no detrusor activity during filling phase and no leakage on coughing. The maximum bladder capacity was 400 ml. Bladder filling was painful. Cystoscopy was normal.

What is the likely diagnosis?

A. Detrusor overactivity
B. Painful bladder syndrome/ sensory urgency
C. Interstitial cystitis
D. Recurrent UTI
E. Endometriosis

81. A 40-year-old woman suffers from dysuria, severe frequency, nocturia and urgency. She also complains of pain or pressure in the suprapubic area. She has been treated with antibiotics for suspected UTI in the past by her GP. On 3 occasions, MSU revealed 'mixed growth'. She has deep dyspareunia and the pain persists for a few days after intercourse. Bladder capacity is around 400 ml. Initial cystoscopy was normal but on repeat filling, some petechial haemorrhage was seen.

What is the most likely diagnosis?

A. Detrusor overactivity
B. Painful bladder syndrome/ sensory urgency
C. Interstitial cystitis
D. Recurrent UTI
E. Endometriosis

82. A 37 year old woman who had 4 vaginal deliveries out of which 1 was a difficult forceps delivery followed by a 3rd degree perineal tear. She presents for the first time with symptoms of Stress

urinary incontinence and on clinical examination incontinence is demonstrated on coughing.

What would be the choice of investigation/ test on her first visit?

A. Urodynamic investigation
B. MSU, culture and sensitivity
C. ultrasound urinary system/KUB
D. Residual urinary volume
E. Pelvic floor muscle tone clinical assessment

83. A woman does not have symptoms of UTI but tests positive for both leucocytes & nitrites on urine dipstick at first visit.

What should be the appropriate management?

A. Treat with antibiotics
B. Send MSU – c/s & prescribe antibiotics only if culture is positive
C. Do not send MSU – c/s
D. Prescribe antibiotics pending culture results
E. Repeat urine dipstix

84. Preferred 2nd line investigation for women with symptoms of voiding difficulty after bladder scan is:

A. Cystoscopy
B. Catheterization post void for residual volume
C. Palpable bladder on Bimanual palpation post void
D. Voiding cystometry
E. MRI bladder

85. A 35-year-old woman presents to urogynaecology clinic with predominantly urinary symptoms.

Cystoscopy should be booked if

A. Previous pelvic cancer
B. Previous pelvic radiation
C. Previous continence surgery

D. Voiding problems
E. Persistent bladder pain

86. A 64-year-old woman who has four normal deliveries presents to clinic with a history of leaking urine on coughing, sneezing. On examination, she has demonstrable stress incontinence. She does not give history of any other urinary symptoms.

The following is the next step in management:

A. Sling surgery
B. Urodynamic Study
C. Tolteradine
D. Bladder scan
E. Bladder drill

87. An elderly woman with cognitive disability and limited mobility is distressed with frequent bedding and clothing changes due to urinary incontinence contamination.

The preferred management plan would be:

A. Intermittent self-catheterization
B. Indwelling catheter
C. Suprapubic catheterization
D. Intraurethral devices to prevent leakage
E. Muscarinic receptor antagonist

88. An 80-year-old hypertensive lady has Overactive bladder symptoms.

The single best option for drug therapy:

A. Oxybutinin (immediate release)
B. Darifenacin
C. Detrusitol
D. Vaginal oestrogen
E. Imipramine

89. A 45-year-old woman with OAB diagnosed clinically is put on oxybutynin tablets but is unable to tolerate the medicines after 4 weeks. The next step would be

A. Change to alternative medications eg. Tolteradine
B. Change to transdermal medication
C. Change to Imipramine
D. Change to Mirabegron
E. Refer to MDT
F. Change to Desmopressin

90. A 35-year-old woman present with painful micturition and increased frequency and nocturia. A provisional diagnosis of interstitial cystitis is made.

Most definitive feature in bladder biopsy in Insterstitial cystitis

A. Normal
B. Mast cells
C. Increased autoimmune antibodies
D. Hypertrophic cells
E. Transitional cell metaplasia

91. A 30-year-old lady complains of persistent leakage of flatus and faeces. She had a complex forceps delivery for an Occipito posterior position when she and a 3B perineal tear. Pelvic floor exercises have not helped.

The next management option is:

A. Ano rectal manometry
B. EMG
C. Pudendalnerve conduction studies
D. Anal mucosal sensitivity testing
E. Endo anal ultrasound

92. A 19-year-old sexually active woman with history of 3 termination of pregnancies. She normally uses Combined oral contraceptive pills but admits to missing pills on occasions. She gives a history of using

condoms regularly. She had been to the GUM clinic and had been treated for Chlamydia and Gonorrhoea in the past.

What contraceptive advice should be given?

A. Depo Medroxy Progesterone Acetate
B. Combined oral Contraceptive Pills
C. Copper IUCD
D. Mirena IUS
E. Progesterone only pill

93. A 18-year-old woman presents with a history of postcoital bleeding for the last two months. She has been in a relationship for three months and is taking the combined oral contraceptive.

The most appropriate investigation is:

A. Transvaginal ultrasound scan
B. Cervical cytology
C. Colposcopy
D. High vaginal swab
E. Endocervical swab

94. A 23-year-old woman presents with a history of pelvic pain and deep dyspareunia for the past 5 months. She and her partner received treatment for Chlamydia six months ago.

The most appropriate investigation is:

A. Transvaginal ultrasound scan
B. Cervical cytology
C. High vaginal swab
D. Endocervical swab
E. Laparoscopy

95. A 22-year-old woman has presented to A&E giving a history of sexual assault involving vaginal intercourse.

Which of the following investigation is NOT necessary?

A. Vulval swab
B. Perineal swab
C. Rectal swab
D. Swab from the speculum
E. Swab from lubricant

96. A 4-year-old child has been found to have sexually transmitted disease. On questioning, history is suggestive of child abuse.

Which of the following disease is not sexually transmitted?

A. Gonorrhoea
B. Syphilis
C. Herpes simplex
D. Chlamydia
E. HIV (Did not have congenital HIV)

97. A 28-year-old woman presents to the family planning clinic and wants combined contraceptive pills for contraception. She is prescribed microgynon and is being counselled regarding venous thromboembolism (VTE) risks of the pill.

What is her VTE risk?

A. 3:100,000 women/year
B. 10-15:100,000 women/year
C. 20:100,000 women /year
D. 50:100,000 women/year
E. 25: 100,000 women/year

98. A 30-year-old woman who has a 2-month-old infant whom she is breast-feeding presents to the family planning clinic requesting contraceptive pills.

Which one of the following is not a contraindication for her?

A. Has Active hepatic disease
B. Have Recurrent follicular cyst in ovary
C. Has Undiagnosed vaginal bleeding

D. Is on Broad spectrum antibiotics
E. Is on Carbamazepine for epilepsy

99. A 29 year old with BMI of 32 kg/m2 Para 1 who delivered normally 9 months ago has presented to the gynaecology clinic requesting sterilization.

The gynaecologist should avoid doing the procedure because:

A. She took the decision during lactational amenorrhoea 6 months post delivery
B. She is less than 30 years of age
C. She has only one young child
D. She has multiple sexual partners
E. She has a BMI of 32 kg/m2

100. A 40-year-old woman wants permanent method of sterilization. Regarding hysteroscopic sterilization (Essure in UK), the following is true:

A. It should not be done in less than 35 years of age
B. The insert is made of silicon
C. Transvaginal ultrasound is preferred 3 months post procedure
D. Hysterosalpingogram is suggested 3 months post procedure
E. The mechanism is mechanical blockage of the tube

101. An 18-year-old girl has presented to family planning clinic requesting emergency contraception.

The following is true:

A. Levonelle can be given upto 5 days (120 hours) after intercourse
B. Ella One can be given upto 5 days (120 hours) after intercourse
C. Copper IUCD can be used upto 3 days (72 hours) after intercourse
D. All are equally effective in preventing pregnancy if used properly
E. Failure rate is 1-2/100 women year

102. A 47-year-old lady who stopped her period 7 months ago has history of migraines while on the contraceptive pill. She presents with

severe menopausal symptoms mainly vasomotor symptoms and low mood.

What is the best choice of HRT for her?

A. Continuous combined HRT
B. Oestrogen patches
C. Mirena IUS
D. Oestradiol implant
E. Sequential combined therapy

103. A 35-year-old lady is amenorrhoic for the last 6 months and before that her periods were infrequent. She has been experiencing some hot flushes and night sweats. She has no medical problems and is otherwise fit and healthy.

Which one of the following fact is true about premature ovarian failure?

A. A single blood test showing elevated FSH is sufficient for diagnosis
B. Anti-mullerian hormone test is compulsory for diagnosis
C. HRT will act as a contraceptive as she is not having periods
D. She can be offered contraceptive pill or HRT, unless contraindicated.
E. Her risk of breast cancer is the same as postmenopausal women using HRT

104. A 45-year-old multiparous lady undergoes endometrial ablation for menorrhagia.

The following is a common complication of the procedure

A. Infection
B. Vaginal discharge
C. Uterine perforation
D. Thrombosis
E. Haemorrhage

105. A 32-year-old lady presented with soreness of vulva and superficial dyspareunia. On examination of the vulva there are erosive lesions and a diagnosis of lichen planus is made.

Which fact is true about lichen planus?

A. Topical steroids are safe to use in pregnancy and breast-feeding
B. Topical calcineurin inhibitors are safe to use in pregnancy
C. Retinoids are safe to use in pregnancy
D. There is no risk of development of cancer
E. Azathioprine may be beneficial.

106. A 27-year-old lady presented to labour ward at 20 weeks in her 1st pregnancy with lower abdominal pain a trans vaginal ultrasound showed cervical length of 15mm. She has no history of note.

What is her treatment option?

A. Prophylactic vaginal progesterone
B. Prophylactic cervical cerclage
C. Prophylactic cerclage and vaginal progesterone
D. Treatment with vaginal clindamycin
E. Treatment with oral clindamycin

107. A 33-year-old lady primiparous presents at 34 weeks gestation to labour ward with a history of gush of fluid per vaginum. This was confirmed on speculum examination.

Which test best confirms chorioamnionitis?

A. C-reactive protein 20 +WBC of 15
B. White blood cell counts 16+ temperatures 37.7° C
C. Temperature 37.7° C
D. Offensive discharge
E. Fetal tachycardia

108. A 35 year old lady who has raised BMI of 35 kg/m2 and is Type 2 diabetic on Gliclizide, ramipril and simvastatin. She wants to get pregnant and has come to your clinic for pre-pregnancy counselling.

Which of one of the following is the correct advice?

A. Continue ramipril
B. Continue simvastatin
C. Gliclizide is safe to use in pregnancy
D. Advice her to keep her HBA1c level below 48mmol/l
E. Advice her to take folic acid 400micro gram to reduce the risk of neural tube defects

109. A 25-year-old lady was seen by her community midwife at home with complains of feeling unwell with pyrexia and rigors. She had an instrumental delivery three days ago. She had an episiotomy that was sutured and she is taking regular paracetamol for pain relief but no other complications.

What should prompt an urgent referral to the hospital?

A. Pyrexia of 37.6°C
B. Tachycardia of 85-90beats/min
C. Respiratory rate of more than 20 breaths/ min
D. Abdominal pain
E. Unable to breast-feed.

110. A 33-year-old lady presented to Accident and emergency department with abdominal pain and heavy lochia after a vaginal delivery two days ago. On examination her temperature was 38.5°C, her pulse was 120 beats per minute and her respiratory rate was 25 breaths per minute. On palpation she had a tender uterus.

What is the most appropriate immediate management?

A. Broad spectrum antibiotics
B. Evacuation of retained products of conception
C. IV fluids
D. IV immunoglobulin
E. IV paracetamol

111. A 34-year-old woman presented to Labour ward 2 days after a normal vaginal delivery in the birth centre. She complained of fever and rigors with abdominal pain. A diagnosis of pueperal sepsis was made.

Which statement regarding antibiotics is true?

A. Broad spectrum antibiotics should be administered within 2 hours of suspicion of sepsis
B. Co-amoxiclav covers MRSA
C. Clindamycin covers most streptococci, staphylococci
D. Piperacillin covers MRSA
E. Piperacillin covers ESBL

112. A 32-year-old lady who is 25 weeks pregnant in her second pregnancy comes in contact with a child who has developed chicken pox. She is not immune to chicken pox.

Which one of the following statement is true?

A. VZIG is effective when given upto15 days after exposure.
B. They are potentially infectious from day 8-28 days after exposure if they receive VZIG
C. They are potentially infective from day 8-28days after exposure if they do not receive VZIG
D. A second dose of VZIG may be required if a further exposure is reported within 2 weeks of exposure
E. VZIG can be given even if the patient has developed chicken pox

113. A 32-year-old lady in her second pregnancy presents to antenatal clinic at 22 weeks gestation with genital Herpes. She has never had herpes in the past.

Which of the following is true about counseling her

A. A caesarean section is indicated for delivery
B. Aciclovir is licensed to be used in pregnancy
C. Patient should be referred to fetal medicine

D. Daily suppressive aciclovir from 36 weeks gestation reduces HSV lesions at term
E. Treatment should be delayed till diagnosis is confirmed

114. A 34-year-old lady in her first pregnancy has had recurrent attacks of herpes this year. She is 20weeks pregnant and seen in antenatal clinic.

Which one of the following statement is true about her further management?

A. Aciclovir is licensed to use in pregnancy
B. She will need a caesarean section
C. Risk of Neonatal herpes is low even if lesions are present at the time of delivery
D. Standard suppressive dose of aciclovir is 400mg twice a day
E. There is increased risk of preterm labour, preterm rupture of membranes

115. A 27-year-old lady in her second pregnancy had her booking bloods done and she has positive treponomal serology. She is then admitted to the antenatal ward for treatment.

Which one of the following is correct?

A. The rate of Jarisch-Herxheimer reaction is 5%
B. The rate of Jarisch-Herxheimer reaction is 20%
C. The rate of Jarisch-Herxheimer reaction is 40%
D. The rate of Jarisch-Herxheimer reaction is 60%
E. The rate of Jarisch-Herxheimer reaction is 10%

116. A 32-year-old multiparous woman presents to antenatal clinic at 37 weeks' gestation with breech presentation on ultrasound scan. She is counselled for external cephalic version (ECV).

Which one of the following conditions is a relative contraindication for the patient to have ECV?

A. Ante–partum haemorrhage
B. Multiple pregnancy
C. Placenta praevia
D. Previous Caesarean section
E. Ruptured membranes

117. A 33-year-old woman with insulin dependent diabetes mellitus presents to the antenatal clinic at 7 weeks. She wants to know about the risks to her baby.

Which of the following is not associated with diabetes?

A. Caudal regression syndrome
B. cystic hygroma
C. holoprosencephaly
D. ventricular septal defect
E. Transposition of great vessels

118. A 30-year old multigravida with a clinically big baby has delivered the head of the baby but there is difficulty in delivering the shoulders. Her labour was prolonged. The emergency buzzer is going off.

Which of the following is an appropriate manoeuvre in these clinical emergencies?

A. Bracht manoeuvre
B. Woodscrew manoeuvre
C. Lovset Manoeuvre
D. Leopold manoeuvre
E. Zavanelli Manoeuvre

119. A 45-year lady attends the colposcopy clinic with a high-grade dyskaryosis on smear. She is para 5 and comes to the clinic with her 12-year-old daughter. She does not speak any English but her daughter does speak good English but is scared to stay for the procedure.

What is the most appropriate thing to do?

A. Use her daughter to interpret
B. Reschedule the appointment and book a professional interpreter
C. Continue with consultation

D. See if any staff that is available that speaks her language
E. Speak slowly and simple language and see if the lady understands

120. A 25-year-old lady comes to your antenatal clinic with her husband. She is 20weeks pregnant in her second pregnancy. She had a 4.6kg baby delivered by forceps in Pakistan 5 years ago. She described to midwife who can understand her language that the baby's shoulder got stuck at time of delivery. She does not speak any English and her partner speaks limited English. She is keen to have a vaginal delivery

What is the most appropriate thing to do?

a. Use her husband to interpret
b. Reschedule the appointment and book a professional interpreter
c. Continue with consultation
d. See if any staff that is available that speaks her language
e. Speak slowly and simple language and see if the lady and her partner understands

121. A 23-year-old nulliparous lady presented with chronic pelvic pain, an ultrasound scan showed a 4cm endometrioma on her right ovary.

What is the best management option?

A. Tricycling of combined oral contraceptive pill
B. Ovarian cyst drainage
C. Oophorectomy
D. Ovarian cystectomy
E. Ovarian Drilling

122. A 34-year-old lady is seen by her GP as she is hypothyroid on thyroxine and soon wants to start a family

Which of the following statement is true about physiological changes in pregnancy

a. Decreased levels of thyroxine-binding globulin
b. Reduced clearance of thyroxine-binding globulin
c. Decreased glomerular filtration rate
d. Deceased clearance of free thyroid hormones
e. Decreased clearance of Iodine.

123. A 34 year old lady in her first pregnancy has hypothyroidism and is on Levothyroxine 125ugm/day and is seen in the combined endocrine clinic at 13 weeks gestation.

In what increment should thyroxine be adjusted?

a. 5 μg
b. 15 μg
c. 25 μg
d. 50 μg
e. 35 μg

124. A 32-year-old lady with a history of migraine presents to her GP at 32 weeks of pregnancy with headache.

Which signs or symptoms will suggest Migraine attack?

A. Bilateral
B. Rapid time to peak headache intensity
C. Abnormal neurological examination
D. Pulsating headache
E. Neck stiffness

125. A 35-year-old lady has been referred by her GP with intractable headache of sudden onset.

What is the radiation risk to the fetus by a computed tomography?

a. <0.005 mGy
b. <0.05mGy
c. <0.5 mGy
d. 5.0 mGy
e. 15 mGy

126. A 32-year-old lady at 36 weeks gestation presents with headache of acute onset not relieved with paracetamol.

Which is the imaging modality of choice to exclude cerebral venous thrombosis

a. CT Scan
b. MRI
c. MRV
d. X -ray Head
e. Cranial USS

127. A 25-year-old lady complains of intractable headache. She had a normal delivery 1 day ago and had epidural in labour.

What is the incidence of dural puncture after epidurals?

A. 0.5-2.5%
B. 2.5-5%
C. 5-10%
D. 10-15%
E. 15-20%

128. A 26 year old is having epidural for pain relief in labour. The anaesthetist talks about risks of dural puncture.

What is the incidence of post dural puncture headache if there is accidental dural puncture?

a. 30-40%
b. 40-50%
c. 50-60%
d. 60-70%
e. 70-80%

129. A 30-year-old lady in her second pregnancy has anterior placenta praevia. She has had a previous caesarean section. Ultrasound reveals placenta accreta.

At what gestation should the delivery be planned?

A. 34-35 weeks gestation

B. 38-39 week's gestation
C. 37-38 week's gestation
D. 36-37 week's gestation
E. 39-40 week's gestation

130. A 25-year-old lady in her first pregnancy has vasa praevia at her 20 week scan which was confirmed by transvaginal scan.

What would be her further management?

a. Admission to Hospital
b. MRI scans to confirm diagnosis
c. Deliver by caesarean section at 36 weeks
d. Rescan in third trimester
e. Refer to tertiary centre

131. A 25-year-old lady in her first pregnancy has vasa praevia at her 20 week scan which was confirmed by transvaginal scan.

What is the incidence of the vasa praevia resolving?

A. 5%
B. 10%
C. 15%
D. 20%
E. 25%

132. A 25-year-old lady in her first pregnancy has vasa praevia at her 32 week scan which was confirmed by transvaginal scan. She has not had any vaginal bleeding.

At what gestation should she be delivered?

A. Deliver immediately
B. 33-35 weeks
C. 35-37 weeks
D. 37-39 weeks
E. 39-41 weeks

133. A 32-year-old lady in her second pregnancy is seen in the antenatal clinic at 16 weeks pregnancy. Her booking bloods show presence of anti K antibodies.

What will be the next step in management?

A. Review her after 20 week scan
B. Refer to fetal medicine
C. Repeat bloods at 28 weeks gestation
D. Repeat bloods in 6 weeks
E. E repeats bloods in 2 weeks

134. A 32-year-old lady in her second pregnancy is seen in the antenatal clinic at 16 weeks pregnancy. Her booking bloods show presence of anti c antibodies. The antibody level titre is 8iu/ml

What will be the next step in management?

A. Review her after 20 week scan
B. Refer to fetal medicine
C. Repeat bloods at 28 weeks gestation
D. Repeat bloods in 6 weeks
E. Repeat bloods in 2 weeks

135. A diagnostic test is applied to 1800 women to assess susceptibility to obstetric cholestasis. The prevalence of Obstetric Cholestasis (OC) is 1%.

	OC Present	OC Absent
Test Positive	70	345
Test Negative	40	1345

The false positive rate is:

A. 21%
B. 22%
C. 19%
D. 23%
E. 25%

136. A diagnostic test is applied to 1800 women to assess susceptibility to obstetric cholestasis. The prevalence of Obstetric Cholestasis (OC) is 1%.

	OC Present	OC Absent
Test Positive	70	345
Test Negative	40	1345

The false negative rate is:

A. 35%
B. 37%
C. 36%
D. 34%
E. 31%

137. A 43 year old had colposcopy and cervical biopsy for CIN2 on cytology. The biopsy was mislabeled with another patient's name. The biopsy showed microinvasive cancer.

What would be the next step of management?

A. Complete risk management form and initiate investigation
B. Inform the colposcopy lead consultant
C. Telephone both the patients and explain the problem
D. Write to pathology lab
E. Correct the mistake yourself

138. A 32 year old lady in her second pregnancy presents to her GP at 20 weeks gestation. Her 4 year old son has been diagnosed with chicken pox two days ago. She has never had chicken pox and blood tests shows that she is not immune to chicken pox and has been given VZIG by her GP.

For how long should she be treated as potentially infectious?

A. 1-7 days after exposure
B. 8-21 days after exposure

C. 8-28 days after exposure
D. 8-14 days after exposure
E. 14-21 days after exposure

139. A 34 year old lady presents to her GP at 23 weeks gestation in her first pregnancy with chicken pox rash, which developed this morning. She is pyrexial but otherwise feels well.

What will be the next step in her management?
A. Paracetamol
B. Diclofenac
C. VZIG
D. Intravenous Aciclovir
E. Oral Aciclovir

140. A 23 year old lady at 22weeks gestation is referred by her GP with flu like symptoms and temperature of 39°C with chills and rigors. She has recently returned from Nigeria after visiting her family.

Which one of the following will rule out a diagnosis of Malaria?

A. Single negative blood film within 24 hours
B. Two negative blood film 12- 24 hours apart
C. Three negative blood film 12-24 hours apart
D. A negative rapid antigen test
E. Two rapid antigen test 12- 24 hours apart

141. A 34 year old lady with monochorionic diamniotic twin pregnancy presents to Day Assessment Unit with reduced fetal movements. Ultrasound scan showed fetal demise of one twin.

What is the incidence of intrauterine death of the second twin?

A. 0.2%
B. 2%
C. 12%
D. 22%
E. 32%

142. A 34 year old lady with monochorionic diamniotic twin pregnancy presents to Day Assessment Unit with reduced fetal movements. Ultrasound scan showed fetal demise of one twin.

What is the incidence of neurological abnormality in the second twin?

A. 0.8%
B. 8%
C. 18%
D. 28%
E. 38%

143. A 26 year old lady presents to labour ward with abdominal pain mainly on the right side and nausea at 20 weeks gestation. On examination she is tender on the right side of her abdomen. She has a white cell count of 14×10^9/L. Her ultrasound scan is inconclusive.

What would be the next step in her management?

A. Laparotomy
B. Laparoscopy
C. CT Scan
D. MRI
E. Repeat Ultrasound.

144. A 40 year old lady is having a caesarean section for placenta praevia. You are consenting her in the antenatal clinic.

What is her risk of having a hysterectomy?

A. 1in 100
B. 5 in 100
C. 11in 100
D. 15 in 100
E. 21 in 100

145. A 41 year old lady 36 weeks gestation presents to labour ward with chest pain. An ECG is performed.

Which of the following ECG changes in not a normal variation in pregnancy?

a. 15-20 degrees left axis shift
b. ST Segment depression
c. T wave inversion in inferior and lateral leads
d. ST elevation
e. Q wave in lead ADF

146. A 26 year lady delivered 10 days ago is behaving abnormally since yesterday. She is having hallucinations and is concerned about the baby. She has a supportive family and they report that her behaviour has changed suddenly.

What should the community midwives action be?

A. Refer her to GP
B. Urgent referral to mother and baby unit
C. Urgent referral to A&E
D. Visit her again tomorrow
E. Telephone consultation with her tomorrow

147. A 34 year old lady in her first pregnancy has had recurrent attacks of herpes this year. She is 20 weeks pregnant and you see her in antenatal clinic.

What would be the further management?

A. Daily suppressive therapy aciclovir 400 mg TDS from 36 weeks
B. Daily suppressive therapy aciclovir 400 mg TDS from 24 weeks
C. Daily suppressive therapy aciclovir 400 mg BD from 36 weeks
D. Aciclovir 400mg TDS for 5 day
E. Daily suppressive therapy aciclovir 200mg TDS from 36 weeks.

148. A 36 year old lady presents to labour ward at 24 weeks gestation with abdominal pain. A HVS and MSU has shown group B streptococcus.

What is her further management?

A. IV antibiotics in labour
B. Does not need IV antibiotics in labour
C. Oral antibiotics now and IV antibiotics in labour
D. Oral antibiotics
E. Repeat HVS

149. A 25 year old lady has β thalassemia and is seen in the pre – pregnancy clinic.

Which of the following advice is true?

A. Deferiprone is safe to use in pregnancy
B. Desferrioxamine is safe to use in first trimester.
C. They can continue chelation agent in first trimester pregnancy
D. Serum fructosamine concentrations is a reliable of glycaemic control
E. HbA1c is a reliable marker of glycaemic control

150. A 34 year old lady in her second pregnancy is seen in the Antenatal clinic at 18 weeks gestation with a cervical length of 21 mm. She has history of preterm pre labour rupture of membranes in her last pregnancy.

What is her best management option?

A. Prophylactic vaginal progesterone
B. Prophylactic cervical cerclage
C. Prophylactic cervical cerclage and vaginal progesterone
D. Treatment with antibiotics
E. Rescan for cervical length in 2 weeks.

151. A 26 year old lady is going to work abroad for three months. She is currently 12 weeks pregnant and is enquiring about vaccination.

Which of these vaccinations is contraindicated in pregnancy?

A. Inactivated influenza vaccine
B. Pertussis (whooping cough) vaccine
C. Inactivated polio vaccine
D. Diphtheria toxoid
E. Mumps

152. A 36 year old lady with β thalassemia with a history of splenectomy is seen in the Antenatal Clinic at 12 weeks gestation. Her platelet count is 400x 10^{9}/l.

Which one of following is true about thromboprophylaxis?

A. Low dose Aspirin
B. Low molecular weight Heparin
C. Low dose Aspirin and Low molecular weight Heparin
D. No thromboprophylaxis
E. Clopidogrel

153. A 30 year old primigravida is seen in the antenatal clinic and complains of not feeling happy with the pregnancy and worried that something bad may happen. She keeps on reminding herself of the troubles her mother had when she was pregnant with her younger sibling.

What is the most common mental health problem in pregnancy?

A. Tocophobia
B. Schizophrenia
C. Depression and anxiety
D. Panic attack
E. Bipolar disorder

154. A 30 year old woman is seen on the postnatal ward very confused and hallucinating of seeing a monster trying to take her baby away. She is unable to sleep and goes through stages where she feels low and at other times when she feels agitated.

This is true about psychosis in pregnancy:

A. It can get worse in pregnancy but unlikely to get worse in the postnatal period
B. Affects 1 to 2 % of pregnant women in postnatal period
C. Bipolar disorder is not a risk factor

D. Valproate is safe to treat mental health problems in pregnancy and breast feeding women
E. Can present for the first time in the postpartum period in women with no psychiatric history

155. A 33 year old woman is seen in the antenatal clinic at 10 weeks gestation. This is her second pregnancy and had an uncomplicated labour and delivery for her first baby. She is on Lithium for a severe mental health problem and wishes to have home birth. She is in clinic to discuss her medication.

She should be informed that:

A. The lithium should be stopped gradually
B. The lithium should be stopped in 2nd trimester
C. She should stop lithium immediately
D. She should stop the drug in the third trimester
E. The risk of anomalies will be completely removed when it is stopped

156. A 26 year old woman in her first pregnancy was diagnosed with gestational diabetes at 29 weeks. She is now 36 weeks and has come to discuss mode and timing of delivery.

This is correct about her delivery:

A. Offer induction of labour at 38 weeks if she is diet controlled and the BMs are well controlled.
B. Offer induction of labour at 40+4 weeks if she is diet controlled and the BMs are well controlled
C. Offer induction at 36 weeks if on metformin
D. Offer elective caesarean section at 38 weeks if on metformin and insulin
E. Offer steroids at 36 weeks and induction at 38 weeks if on metformin and insulin.

157. A 26 year old woman in her first pregnancy was diagnosed with gestational diabetes at 29 weeks. She is now 4 weeks postpartum and wants to discuss further monitoring.

Which one of the following is correct?

A. Offer a 75gm 2hour oral glucose tolerance test 6-12 weeks postpartum
B. Offer HBA1c in all women with gestational diabetes at 6 weeks postnatal check
C. Yearly random blood glucose
D. Yearly fasting blood glucose
E. Offer a 50gm oral glucose tolerance test 6 – 12 weeks postpartum

158. A 34 year old woman G3P2 wishes to discuss testing for gestational diabetes.
She should be offered screening if she

A. Has a BMI of 30
B. Has a cousin with type 1 diabetes mellitus
C. Her last baby weighed 4.4kg and the first one weighed 3.9kg
D. Had gestational diabetes in her first pregnancy but not in the second pregnancy
E. Glycosuria of 1+ on one occasion

159. A 27 year old Type 1 diabetic is seen in the diabetic antenatal clinic at 35 weeks gestation. Her insulin requirement has increased recently in the pregnancy. This is her second pregnancy and her first delivery was by caesarean section for fetal distress.

Which of the following statements is correct about her care?

A. Monitor capillary glucose every 30 min in labour
B. Sliding scale with Intravenous dextrose and insulin only if BM is consistently above 8mmol/L in labour
C. Sliding scale with IV dextrose and insulin if the BM <4mmol/L in labour
D. Sliding scale with IV dextrose and insulin if the BM >6mmol/L in labour
E. Sliding scale with IV Normal saline and insulin if the BM <4mmol/L in labour

160. A 22 year old G1P0 presents to the maternity triage with no fetal movements for 12 hours. An ultrasound confirms an intrauterine fetal death at 29 weeks gestation.

Her risk of having disseminated intravascular coagulopathy within 4 weeks is:

A. 10%
B. 20%
C. 30%
D. 15%
E. 5%

161. A 22 year old G1P0 presents to the maternity triage with no fetal movements for 12 hours. An ultrasound confirms an intrauterine fetal death (IUFD) at 29 weeks gestation.

Which infections should she not be screened for, as they are not associated with IUFD?

A. Cytomegalovirus
B. Parvo virus
C. Listeria
D. Toxoplasmosis
E. Mumps

162. A 19 year old lady who had a stillbirth at 38 weeks has come to see you 2 weeks after delivery. She has agreed to have a post-mortem

What percentage of stillbirths has congenital anomalies?

A. 15%
B. 6%
C. 2%
D. 10%
E. 20%

163. A 40 year old G1P0 is unfortunately diagnosed as having an intrauterine fetal death at 40 weeks and 1 day. Cervical examination

shows a bishop score of 2. She is very worried about the side effects of the method of induction of labour.

What is the most cost effective method of induction?

A. Misoprostol
B. Propess
C. Prostin
D. Gemeprost
E. Balloon catheter

164. A 29 year old G3P2 is admitted to labour ward for induction of labour following an intrauterine fetal death at 38 weeks. Her vaginal swab shows Group B streptococcus (GBS). She is worried about infection and ask you when and what antibiotics will be given if needed.

Which of the following is correct?

A. Ciprofloxacin if urinary tract infection is suspected
B. Broad spectrum antibiotics if sepsis is suspected
C. Intrapartum antibiotics if she has a previous child affected by Group B streptococcus
D. Intrapartum benzylpenicillin
E. Routine antibiotic prophylaxis in labour

165. A 33 year old woman with previous uncomplicated caesarean section is having induction of labour at 37 weeks for obstetric cholestasis. She has an epidural and has been complaining of constant pain along the scar for the last hour.

The following may be signs of a scar rupture:

A. Maternal pyrexia
B. Gush of meconium liqour
C. Fetal head sliding up
D. Anuria
E. Epigastric pain

166. A woman brings her baby to the hospital a few days after delivery for hearing assessment. The test shows that the baby has sensory neural hearing loss. She also has microcephaly, hepatosplenomegaly and a rash on the trunk. Blood test showed low platelets. Further test shows that baby has a Patent Ductus Arteriosus. On questioning she mentioned that she had a bad flu earlier in the pregnancy.

The most like cause of the congenital illness is:

A. Cytomegalovirus
B. Syphilis
C. Toxoplasmosis
D. Rubella
E. Varicella

167. A pregnant woman suffering from migraine is seen in the antenatal clinic at 15 weeks gestation. She comes to the clinic after reading a lot about the condition on the Internet. She has noted some of the key points and wants to discuss them with you.

Which of the following statements about migraine will you agree with her?

A. The headache is usually bilateral
B. Pregnancy can lead to a reduction in frequency and severity of attacks
C. There is a 5 fold increase risk of pre eclampsia compared with women without migraine in pregnancy
D. The risk of having a stroke is similar to the risk of having myocardial infarction in pregnant women suffering from migraine.
E. Initial first line treatment is usually amitriptyline

168. A 27 year old woman with a prolonged labour has now reached full dilatation and been pushing for the last 2 hours. She has not delivered and you decide to take her to theatre for a trial of instrumental delivery or caesarean section. She is worried about the effects of instrumental delivery and /or caesarean section at second stage

Which of the following statements are correct?

A. There is increased risk of hemorrhoids with instrumental delivery

B. Women who have operative vaginal delivery compared to caesarean section are less likely to report difficulties conceiving
C. Consultant presence has not been shown to reduce caesarean section rates at second stage
D. Constipation is more common following operative vaginal delivery compared to following caesarean section at second stage at about a year following delivery.
E. There is evidence that the risk of maternal morbidity is higher for caesarean section after an unsuccessful forceps delivery compared to an unsuccessful ventouse delivery.

169. You are leading a skills and drills session for Senior House Officers and midwifes and discussing management of Post Partum Haemorrhage (PPH)

Which of these statements is correct?

A. Carbetocin is not licensed in the UK although used effectively for PPH prophylaxis
B. Oxytocics reduces risk of PPH by 40%
C. Intravenous access must be obtained with a 12 gauge cannula
D. Oxytocics reduces risk of PPH by 80%
E. Oxytocics reduces risk of PPH by 60%

170. A 41 year old woman attends the antenatal clinic at 28 weeks gestation as part of her regular antenatal clinic visits. She is HIV positive on combined antiretroviral therapy. Her CD4 count is 450cells /μl and viral load <50copies /ml.

What is the estimated Mother to Child Transmission (MTCT) in such a woman in UK?

A. 0.17%
B. 1%
C. 1.2%
D. 0.57%
E. 0.2%

171. A 30 year old woman HIV positive mother of one presents as a late booker to the antenatal clinic. She is 28 weeks pregnant, well and is not on any medications for her HIV. Her viral load is < 50copies /ml and CD4 count 450cells /μl

The following statement is correct about her management:

A. She can be started on zidovudine monotherapy
B. She can be started on Abacavir monotherapy
C. She can be started on Lamivudine monotherapy
D. There is evidence that combined antiretroviral therapy is more effective in reducing vaginal viral shedding compared to zidovudine in women with above results
E. It is too late to start any treatment

172. A 24 year old woman who delivered about 8 hours ago is complaining of feeling unwell. Her labour was uncomplicated and this was her first delivery. Her temperature is 39°C, pulse is 120bpm and blood pressure is 90/50mmHg. She has developed a rash on inner part of her left thigh and there is a high suspicion of sepsis.

Which organism is the most likely cause of the sepsis?

A. Streptococcus pneumoniae
B. Staphylococcus aureus
C. Escherichia Coli
D. Streptococcus pyogenes
E. Listeria

173. A woman attends the postnatal perineal clinic to discuss her care and management in her recent delivery. She sustained a third degree tear (3c), which was repaired appropriately in theatre. She has no bowel related symptoms and wants to know if it could have been prevented and the recurrence rate.

Which of the following should she be told?

A. The recurrence rate in subsequent delivery is about 25%

B. The recurrence rate in subsequent delivery is about 20%
C. The incidence of anal sphincter injury after vaginal delivery is about 3%
D. The incidence of anal sphincter injury after vaginal delivery is about 1%
E. The recurrence rate in subsequent deliveries is about 10 %

174. A 30 year old woman in her second pregnancy attends the specialist midwife clinic to discuss vaginal birth after caesarean section. Her first baby was delivered by caesarean section for cord prolapse. The operation was uncomplicated and she is keen on having a vaginal delivery this time.

Which statement is correct?

A. Risk of placenta previa after 2 previous caesarean section is 2%
B. 0.8% risk of scar dehiscence after 1 previous caesarean section
C. 8% risk of scar dehiscence after 2 previous caesarean sections
D. The absolute risk of birth related perinatal death in women having a trial of vaginal birth after caesarean is more than a woman having her first vaginal delivery.
E. Risk of placenta previa after 1 previous caesarean section is 1%

175. A 27 year old woman G1P0 with an uncomplicated pregnancy wishes to discuss the pros and cons of having a home birth.

She should be informed that there is no significant difference in:

A. Blood transfusion rate
B. Vaginal delivery rate
C. Neonatal outcome
D. Episiotomy rate
E. Caesarean section rate

176. A 40 year old woman with a prolonged second stage of labour is having a trial of instrumental delivery.

Compared with vacuum extraction, forceps delivery is

A. More likely associated with cephalheamatoma
B. Less likely associated with maternal trauma
C. More likely associated with the need for phototherapy
D. Less likely associated with the use of multiple instruments
E. More likely to fail

177. A 32 year old lady has dichorionic diamniotic twin pregnancy. The pregnancy was spontaneously conceived and there are no particular problems in the pregnancy. Her growth scans has been normal. She is planning to fly to her mother's house for delivery.

Up to what gestation can she safely fly?

A. 33 weeks
B. 32 weeks
C. 34 weeks
D. 36 weeks
E. 30 weeks

178. A 34 year old primiparous woman is seen in antenatal clinic at 30 weeks. She asks whether she can fly to India in pregnancy.

What are the contraindications for flight travel?

A. She is anemic and her Hb is 7.8g/dl
B. She has history of migraine
C. She suffers from severe asthma
D. She is sickle cell trait
E. She is being investigated for palpitations

179. A 42 year old primigravida is in spontaneous labour at term. She is progressing well with 3:10 regular contractions and is 7 cm dilated. She ruptured her membranes spontaneously 6 hours ago and the liquor is clear. The CTG is pathological. A fetal blood sampling is performed and the fetal lactate is 4.3mmol/l.

What should be the next step of management?

A. Grade 1 caesarean section

B. Grade 2 caesarean section
C. Repeat FBS in 20 mins
D. Repeat FBS in 60 mins
E. Continue labour

180. A 42 year old primigravida is being seen in antenatal clinic at 38 weeks. She has come to discuss timing of delivery. She is being advised to have induction of labour at 40 weeks due to increased risk of stillbirth.

What is the risk of stillbirth at her age?
A. 1.5 in 1000
B. 2 in 1000
C. 1 in 1000
D. 2.5 in 1000
E. 0.5 in 1000

181. A 28 year old primigravida woman has immigrated to UK from Afghanistan. Her Vitamin D levels is 25nmol/l. She should be given Vitamin D supplementation.

The following are the risks associated with maternal hypovitaminosis D:

A. Gestational Diabetes
B. Primary Caesarean Section
C. Candida Infection
D. Fetal Hypoglycemia
E. Maternal Asthma

182. A 32 year old primiparous lady has been induced for postdates. She has progressed to full dilatation with syntocinon infusion. She has been pushing for an hour and is contracting 4: 10. The CTG is pathological and delivery should be expedited. On examination, the vertex is at spines and is in left occipito transverse postion. There is 1+ caput with no moulding. Decision is made to use a posterior cup for delivery.

What is the flexion point at which the cup should be applied?

A. On the sagittal suture 3cm in front of the posterior fontanelle

B. On the sagittal suture 2cm in front of the posterior fontanelle
C. On the sagittal suture 3 cm in front of the anterior fontanelle
D. On the sagittal suture 2cm in front of the anterior fontanelle
E. On the coronal suture 3cm in front of the posterior fontanelle

183. A 39 year old P1 woman is being induced for gestational diabetes at 38 weeks. She is 4 cm dilated and syntocinon is being started after ARM at 3cm following propess insertion. She wants an effective form of analgesia. The anaesthetist has discussed remifentanil PCA.

Which of the following is a characteristic of Remifentanil PCA?
A. It acts within 20 mins of giving the drug
B. 1 in 8 women will require Entonox in addition
C. Continuous fetal monitoring is required
D. There is 1 in 15 risk of failure
E. Regular blood pressure monitoring is required

184. A 32 year old woman, who is 33 weeks pregnant in her second pregnancy, is worried about group B streptococcus infection of her newborn. She is in the antenatal clinic and wants GBS screening.

Intrapartum antibiotics prophylaxis should be offered to women if:

A. GBS screen positive in previous pregnancy
B. GBS bacteriuria (growth>10^2cfu/ml) in current pregnancy
C. During elective caesarean section for breech
D. GBS is detected on vaginal swab taken for whitish vaginal discharge at 12 weeks of pregnancy
E. Preterm rupture of membrane occurs at 33weeks gestation

185. A 28 year old woman with monochorionic diamniotic twins is seen in Foetal Medicine Clinic. She is suspected to have Twin to Twin Transfusion syndrome.

On ultrasound, the following criteria is not necessary for diagnosis:

A. Concordant gender
B. Oligohydramnios in one sac and polyhydramnios in other
C. Discordant bladder

D. Hydrops of one twin
E. Haemodynamic compromise

186. A 32 year old woman has generalised pruritus but no rash. She had obstetrics cholestasis in her previous pregnancy. Routine blood tests are being done 2 weekly to diagnose/ assess obstetrics cholestasis.

The following blood test is not generally helpful in diagnosis of obstetric cholestasis:

A. Alanine transaminases
B. Unconjugated Bilirubin
C. Chenodeoxycholic acid
D. Alkaline phosphatase
E. Gamma glutamyl transpeptidase

187. A 28 year old woman is 28 weeks pregnant in her second pregnancy. She had an elective caesarean section for breech presentation in her previous pregnancy. Her 20 weeks foetal anomaly scan suggested a low-lying placenta covering the internal cervical os. She is being counselled in the antenatal clinic.

The following management plan should be instituted:

A. Transabdominal scan at 32 weeks
B. Transabdominal scan at 36 weeks
C. Transvaginal scan at 32 weeks
D. Transvaginal scan at 36 weeks
E. MRI at 32 weeks

188. A 34 year old woman just had an uncomplicated vaginal delivery. This is her 4th vaginal delivery. Her serum haemoglobin is 8.8g/dl.

The prophylactic oxytocic of choice is:

A. Oxytocin
B. Ergometrine
C. Syntometrine

D. Misoprostol
E. Carbetocin

189. A 28 year old woman presents at 32 weeks gestation with threatened preterm labour. She is being given corticosteroids for foetal lung maturity. Tocolysis is therefore being considered.

The most effective tocolytic (may or may not be licenced in U.K.) is

A. Ritodrine (beta mimetic)
B. Magnesium sulphate
C. Rofecoxib (COX2 inhibitor)
D. Nifedipine (calcium channel blocker)
E. Indomethacin (COX2 inhibitor)

190. A 37 year old woman has presented at 10 weeks gestation. She has a child with Trisomy 21. She wants to discuss screening tests as well as definitive investigations to exclude Chromosomal abnormalities.

While counselling her, the following is not correct about Amniocentesis and CVS:

A. CVS should be performed after 9 weeks gestation
B. Early amniocentesis is associated with a higher risk of talipes
C. Amniocentesis in the 3rd trimester is associated with a significant risk of emergency delivery
D. There is a greater likelihood of multiple attempts if amniocentesis is done in the 3rd trimester
E. Amniocentesis should not be done in women who are Hepatitis C carriers

191. A 35 year old woman is 25 weeks pregnant. There are concerns about foetal wellbeing and a discussion about possible caesarean section and antenatal corticosteroids is being undertaken.

The following is correct about antenatal corticosteroid administration to prevent respiratory distress syndrome in newborn:

A. In Intrauterine growth restriction, should be given between 24 and 34 weeks gestation
B. In twins at increased risk of preterm delivery, given upto 34+6 weeks gestation
C. In any woman at risk of preterm labour upto 34 weeks gestation
D. Should be avoided in overt chorioamnionitis
E. Robust data suggests giving it is particularly effective in preventing neonatal problems between 24-26 weeks

192. A 25 year old woman in her first pregnancy presents at 32 weeks gestation with a second episode of reduced foetal movement. On clinical examination she has a small for gestational age foetus.

The following tests cannot be done to assess:

A. Formal foetal count (Kick chart)
B. Cardio tocogram
C. Biophysical profile
D. Ultrasound scan
E. Computerised Cardiotocogram

193. A 30 year old woman in her second pregnancy is seen in the antenatal clinic at 15weeks gestation. Red cell antibodies have been detected in the booking blood. Her combined serum test for chromosomal anomalies has come back high risk.

In her management, the following should be followed:

A. Amniocentesis is contraindicated
B. Refer to Foetal Medicine unit only if Anti D titres >2IU/ml
C. Refer to Foetal Medicine unit only if Anti c titres > 4IU/ml
D. Refer to Foetal Medicine unit only if Anti K titres > 6IU/ml
E. Refer to Foetal Medicine unit if Anti E and Anti c antibodies are detected

194. A 30 year old Rh (D) negative woman is having an emergency caesarean section for major placenta praevia and heavy antepartum haemorrhage at 30 weeks gestation. She has had her routine antibody testing at 28 weeks, when no antibody was detected and had her

prophylactic Anti D Immunoglobulin. Cell salvage and reinfusion of her blood is done since she is Jehova's witness.

In her treatment, she should have:

A. 500 IU of Anti D Immunoglobulin if cord blood group is D positive
B. 1500 IU of Anti D Immunoglobulin if cord blood group is D positive
C. A Kleihauer done immediately after reinfusion to check if additional Anti D is needed
D. A Kleihauer done 1 hour after reinfusion to check if additional Anti D is needed
E. 500 IU of Anti D Immunoglobulin should be given immediately after reinfusion without any delay to check baby's blood group.

195. A 28 year old woman presents to labour ward 12 hours after a normal uncomplicated vaginal delivery, hypotensive, pyrexial and tachypnoic. Her lactate is 6 mmol/l. She develops severe pain in her lower limbs. Deep vein thrombosis is suspected but Doppler ultrasound is negative.

In her management, the following should be avoided:

A. Broad spectrum antibiotics including Piperacillin, Tazobactam or Carbapenem and Clindamycin
B. Analgesics including NSAIDs
C. Transfer to Intensive Therapy unit
D. Newborn should be given antibiotics irrespective of his/her clinical condition
E. Surgical referral made

196. In the Confidential Enquiry of Maternal Death and Morbidities, 2015, which was the leading indirect cause of maternal death?
A. Cardiac Disease
B. Thrombosis and Thromboembolism
C. Psychiatric Disease
D. Influenza
E. Cancer

197. A 34 year old P2 lady unfortunately sustained a spinal cord injury above T4 level. She has given birth to her 2nd child and is planning to breast feed the baby.

Breast-feeding is affected in the following manner:

A. No affect
B. Delayed
C. Only long term breast feeding is affected
D. Autonomic dysreflexia
E. Increased production of breast milk

198. A 28 year P1 woman is in spontaneous labour. She had a normal delivery in the past and is very keen to have vaginal delivery. She had an uncomplicated pregnancy and was admitted to labour ward in active labour. She ruptured her membranes 2 hours ago and the liquor is clear. She is now 5cm dilated and is contracting 4:10. The CTG has a baseline of 155bpm, variability is 5 – 10 bpm and late decelerations with >50% contractions for 30 mins. FBS was attempted twice (by resident consultant) and this failed. There was acceleration on fetal scalp stimulation.

What should be the next step of management?

A. Caesarean section
B. Repeat attempt at FBS
C. Continue labour
D. Attempt FBS again in 1 hour
E. Start syntocinon to expedite labour

199. A ST3 trainee is being supervised for third degree tear repair of a 26 year old primiparous who sustained a 3rd degree tear during forceps delivery which was also performed by the trainee. The ST3 trainee has done 2 other repairs before this.

Which of the following work placed based assessment tools should be used?

A. Summative OSAT
B. Formative OSAT
C. DOPS
D. Mini CeX
E. CBD (Case based discussion)

200. A 39 year old primiparous woman presented to labour ward with regular contractions – 4 in 10 minutes. On admission, she was 9 cm dilated. She progressed to full dilatation in 2 hours and after 1 hour of passive descent, pushed actively for 1.5 hours. The on call registrar assessed her and the findings were: Cervix – full dilatation; vertex at -1; direct occiputo-posterior postion, caput 2+ and moulding 1+. She was recommended a trial of instrumental +/- emergency caesarean section and was transferred to theatre.

The following statement is true about the impact of a caesarean section

A. Caesarean section at full dilatation has more than 4 times risk of intraoperative trauma compared to CS at first stage of labour
B. The risk of laceration to bladder, bowel and uterine extension is in the range of 10% to 27%
C. Risk of Maternal haemorrhage of >1000mls is more than 20% with 2nd stage CS
D. Clavicle fracture and brachial plexus injury is more common with 2nd stage CS
E. Maternal sepsis and wound infection risk is significantly higher in 2nd stage CS

Chapter 5

ANSWERS AND EXPLANATIONS

EXTENDED MATCHING QUESTIONS (EMQS)

1. C

If a woman is on enzyme inducing drugs, then they should be on other forms of contraception, which is not affected by them such as POP. If they need COCP, then they should have a higher dose such as 50μg ethinylestradiol with a shorter pill free period for 4 days.

2. A

Current Breast cancer is a risk UKMEC risk 4 for COC and POP. If they have remained disease free for 5 years, still it is UKMEC 3.

3. F

Levonorgesterol 1500mg (Levonelle) can only be used for emergency contraception within 72 hours. But Ulipristal acetate 30mg (Ellaone) can be used upto 120 hours, as is copper coil.

4. L

Ideally COC is better to prevent irregular bleeding, however in the presence of 2 relative contraindications – smoking and raised BMI – a newer generation POP such as desogestrol may have less side effects.

5. B

Women who are not breastfeeding can start COC 21 days postpartum.

Ref: Faculty of Sexual Health Clinical Guidance
http://www.fsrh.org/pages/Clinical_Guidance_2.asp

6. I

Single dose first generation cephalosporin or ampicillin IV is the choice of drug for caesarean section to reduce postoperative infection.

7. J

Metronidazole and a broad-spectrum antibiotic should be used at induction for third degree tear repair, manual removal of placenta.

8. L

There is no need for postoperative antibiotics unless there are any significant symptoms suggestive of infection. They should have received intraoperative antibiotics

9. C

For surgical termination of pregnancy metronidazole is necessary for anaerobic cover.

Ref: StratOG Module – Surgical Procedure and Postoperative Care

10. M

If the smear shows mild dyskaryosis, but the High risk HPV is positive, they should be referred for colposcopy for routine follow up in 6 weeks

11. N

Same as above but if the high risk HPV is negative; they can have routine recall in 3 years

12. K

If the first smear is high grade, they should have colposcopy urgently

13. M

3 inadequate smears need referral to colposcopy as routine

14. C

Women who had treatment for high-grade lesion should have cervical smear with HPV testing by the GP

15. E

If the test of cure is negative at 6 months follow up post treatment, they should have repeat yearly smear.

16. I

If the deeper margins continue to have CIN3, then LLETZ should be repeated

17. I

If the margins show CIN even if the cancer area is excised, they should have repeat LLETZ

Ref: NHS Cervical Screening Program (NHSCSP) Guideline No: 20

18. B

Endometrial hyperplasia without atypia i.e. simple hyperplasia should be treated with continuous progesterone. If the patient declines LNG-IUS, she can have oral progesterone.

19. F

Persistent endometrial hyperplasia and symptoms in a raised BMI patient needs a definitive treatment in the form of hysterectomy if the conservative treatment has failed. As she is 43, the ovaries should be conserved.

20. F

As above

21. L

Patients should have endometrial surveillance post treatment with endometrial biopsy every 6 months. If at least 2 biopsies are negative, they can be discharged.

22. N

They should have progesterone therapy and repeat biopsy at the end of 3 months, which should be negative prior to conceiving.

23. A

Women on tamoxifen and with multiple polyps should have LNG-IUS to maintain thin endometrium with endometrial surveillance.

Ref: Management of Endometrial Hyperplasia
Green-top Guideline No. 67

24. J

In outpatient hysteroscopy, the diameter of the hysteroscope is only 2.7mm with 3 – 3.5mm sheath. Hydrodilatation should be performed and the evidence suggests no anesthetic is needed even in a nulliparous woman.

25. D

If operative procedure such as polypectomy is being done, then cervical dilatation is needed and hence paracervical or intracervical block should be given.

26. B

If a tenaculum is used to grasp the cervix, local anaesthetic is the form of topical anesthesia to the ectocervix should be given.

Ref: Best Practice in Outpatient Hysteroscopy
Green-top Guideline No. 59

27. A

Injury to the inferior epigastric artery is one of the known risk factors of lateral port insertion during laparoscopy

28. E

Ureteric injury is one of the risk factor during anterior repair. Especially after the hysterectomy the anatomy of the ureter may be distorted.

29. G

Insertion of the trans obturator tape (TOT) is through the Obturator foramen through which the obturator nerve also passes

30. B

The injury of this nerve is common during extensive pelvic wall surgery

31. J

Risk of pudendal nerve injury is high during sacrospinous fixation.

Ref: Nerve Injuries associated with gynaecological surgeries
TOG 2014, Volume 16, 1
Urinary tract injuries in laparoscopic gynaecological surgery; prevention, recognition and management
TOG 2014, Volume 16, 1

32. A

Woman with BRCA1 mutation has 63% ovarian cancer risk and 85% breast cancer risk by the age of 70.

33. H

Lynch Syndrome related ovarian cancer is usually early stage and moderately or well differentiated. They also have synchronous endometrial cancer more commonly then other ovarian cancers.

34. B

Woman with BRCA2 mutation has 27% ovarian cancer risk and 84% breast cancer risk by the age of 70.

35. E

Mutation of PTEN tumour suppressor gene causes Bannayan-Riley-Ruvalcaba Syndrome in children and Cowden Syndrome in adulthood.

36. F

Peutz-Jeghers Syndrome is an autosomal dominant gastrointestinal polyposis disorder, which confers high risk of gynaecological cancer

37. G

Li-Fraumeni Syndrome is caused by germline mutation of TP53. It puts a patient at high risk of early onset breast cancer and gynaecological cancer mainly epithelial ovarian cancer.

Ref: Management of Women with Genetic Predisposition to Gynaecological Cancers
Scientific Impact Paper No: 48

38. B

Joel-Cohen incision is a straight transverse incision 3cm below the anterior superior iliac spine higher than the Pfanneisteil Incision. It's the most commonly used incision for caesarean section.

39. C

In Maylard Incision, all the layers of the abdomen are incised about 3-8 cm above the symphysis pubis. This would be used in women with history of previous surgeries or where because of patient habitus access is difficult.

40. G

A midline incision is needed in view of the large size of the ovarian cyst. A simple cyst could be deflated through a small incision, however a dermoid cyst is not easy to deflate. Also, efforts should be made to have minimal spillage into the abdomen.

41. J

Gridiron incision of McBurney is used for open appendicectomy

Ref: Abdominal Incisions and Sutures in Obstetrics and Gynaecology TOG 2014, Volume 16, 1

42. D

Tachycardia, tachypnea and pyrexia are signs of sepsis. It can be common after any uterine manipulating surgery

43. A

The symptoms are suggestive of vault hematoma. Women on long-term anticoagulants are at high risk of developing vault hematoma post hysterectomy. Care must be taken to achieve good hemostasis.

44. F

Paralytic ileus is a common complication any abdominal surgery especially if bowel handling has been done during surgery. Careful assessment and investigation should rule out bowel damage. Tympanic or sluggish bowel sounds can both be associated with paralytic ileus. However, in bowel injury, the bowel sounds would be absent.

45. H

Injury to ureter is a common side effect during pelvic surgery. If there is no complete transection of the ureter, there could be an urinoma formation only which can be managed conservatively.

46. E

Lymphorrhea is a common complication of oncological surgery where extensive lymphadenectomy has been performed. The serum biochemistry is the same as in serum whereas it would be different for urine.

47. B

Vesico-vaginal fistula is a rare complication of gynaecological surgery and even rarer in a caesarean section. The woman would complain of continuous urine leakage. It can be diagnosed on a speculum examination. Micturating cystourethrogram is the investigation of choice for confirmed diagnosis.

48. A

	IUGR Present	IUGR Absent
Test Positive	50 (True positive)	200 (False positive)
Test Negative	20 (False negative)	1230 (True negative)

Sensitivity = TP/(TP+FN) = 50/(50+20) = 71.4%

49. H

Specificity = TN/(FP+TN) = 1230/(200+1230) = 86%

50. J

Positive likelihood ratio = sensitivity/ (1- specificity) = (0.71/1- 0.86) = 5.07

51. F

Negative likelihood ration = (1- sensitivity)/specificity = (1-0.71)/0.86 = 0.34

Ref: Statistical Analysis

52. A

For proximal tubal occlusion, hysteroscopic tubal cannulation or selective salpingography and tubal cannulation may be effective if expertise is available, particularly in mild tubal disease

Ref: (NICE CG156: Fertility Problems: Assessment and Treatment)

53. C

Salpingectomy before IVF improves the chances of live birth

Ref: (NICE CG156: Fertility Problems: Assessment and Treatment)

54. H

Amenorrhoea and intrauterine adhesions should be offered hysteroscopic adhesiolysis because this may restore menstruation and fertility

Ref: (NICE CG156: Fertility Problems: Assessment and Treatment)

55. I

Surgical treatment should be offered to women with severe endometriosis. However, where extensive bowel or ureteric resection or colostomy may be needed, it is preferable to proceed to IVF

Ref: (NICE CG156: Fertility Problems: Assessment and Treatment)

56. G

If the male partner is HIV positive, IUI with washed sperms is an option

Ref: (NICE CG156: Fertility Problems: Assessment and Treatment)

57. D

IVF should be offered to couple with unexplained subfertility after trying regularly to conceive for 2 years

Ref: (NICE CG156: Fertility Problems: Assessment and Treatment)

58. B

In women with WHO Type 1 ovulatory failure, pulsatile gonadotrophin releasing hormone or gonadotrophins with LH / HCG activity should be given. However, pulsatile gonadotrophins are logistically difficult because they need to be given frequently

Ref: (NICE CG156: Fertility Problems: Assessment and Treatment)

59. E

Women with WHO Type 2 ovulatory failure and clomiphene resistance (after 6 months of clomiphene) should be offered either clomiphene + metformin or ovarian drilling or gonadotrophins. Gonadotrophins need extensive monitoring and therefore rarely offered in secondary care.

Ref: (NICE CG156: Fertility Problems: Assessment and Treatment)

60. F

She probably has microprolactinoma. Hyperprolactinaemia causing anovulation should be treated with dopamine agonists

Ref: (NICE CG156: Fertility Problems: Assessment and Treatment)

61. D

WHO type 2 ovulatory disorders can be treated with either clomiphene or metformin or both taking into account BMI, ease of use. Since she is type 2 diabetic, metformin is preferred.

Ref: (NICE CG156: Fertility Problems: Assessment and Treatment)

62. G

Women aged between 40-42 should be offered IVF after 2 years of regular unprotected intercourse, provided they never had IVF, there is no evidence of low ovarian reserve and understands the implications of pregnancy at this age.

Ref: (NICE CG156: Fertility Problems: Assessment and Treatment)

63. H

Ref: (NICE CG156: Fertility Problems: Assessment and Treatment)

64. G

Even though the second trimester miscarriage is suspected to be due to cervical incompetence, cervical cerclage, particularly without objective evidence is not without risks.

Ref: (RCOG GTG 17: April2011: The Investigation and Treatment of couples with recurrent 1st trimester and second trimester miscarriages.)

65. L

Aspirin and heparin combination as opposed to aspirin alone reduces the risk by 56% and therefore more effective

Ref: (RCOG GTG 17: April2011: The Investigation and Treatment of couples with recurrent 1st trimester and second trimester miscarriages.)

66. K

Insufficient evidence that either metformin or suppression of high LH levels prevent recurrent miscarriage

Ref: (RCOG GTG 17: April2011: The Investigation and Treatment of couples with recurrent 1st trimester and second trimester miscarriages.)

67. K

Treatment against NK cells and immunotherapy or steroids do not improve live birth rate

Ref: (RCOG GTG 17: April2011: The Investigation and Treatment of couples with recurrent 1st trimester and second trimester miscarriages.)

68. K

Insufficient evidence that HCG or progesterone prevents recurrent miscarriage

Ref: (RCOG GTG 17: April2011: The Investigation and Treatment of couples with recurrent 1st trimester and second trimester miscarriages.)

69. B

For incomplete miscarriage use 600 mcg of single dose misoprostol and for missed miscarriage use 800 mcg of single dose misoprostol.

Ref: (NICE CG 154: Dec, 2012: Ectopic pregnancy and miscarriage: Diagnosis and initial management)

70. A

Medical termination between 9-13 weeks, mifepristone followed by misoprostol 36-48 hours later: 800 mcg vaginally followed by 4 further dosage of 400 mcg each vaginally or orally at 3-4 hourly intervals

Ref: (The care of women requesting Induced Abortion: RCOG CG 7: November, 2011)

71. I

Antibiotic prophylaxis against Chlamydia trachomatis is to be given for both medical and surgical termination of pregnancy. Azithromycin + Metronidazole or Doxycycline + Metronidazole are preferred if chlamydia has not been excluded or positive. If Chlamydia has been tested for preoperatively and negative, only Metronidazole will suffice

Ref: (RCOG GTG 17: April2011: The Investigation and Treatment of couples with recurrent 1st trimester and second trimester miscarriages.)

72. C

NSAID s should be prescribed for pain relief because they are effective. Paracetamol is ineffective and should not be prescribed.

Ref: (RCOG GTG 17: April2011: The Investigation and Treatment of couples with recurrent 1st trimester and second trimester miscarriages.)

73. E

Oxytocics should be avoided until evacuation is complete in gestational trophoblastic disease to reduce the dissemination of trophoblastic tissue in invasive mole.

Ref: (The Management of Gestational Trophoblastic Disease: RCOG GTG: 38; Feb, 2008)

74. B

A thin line of endometrium is seen connecting to the periphery of the interstitial sac. This is called the interstitial line sign. Using 3D ultrasound, a connection is almost always seen with the endometrial cavity.

75. E

The ultrasound features in cervical pregnancy include a barrel shaped cervix, empty uterus, the gestational sac below the level of internal cervical os, a negative sliding sign and a positive Doppler showing sustained peritrophoblastic circulation. These women will often have heavy bleeding but will not pass the products of conception.

76. C

Heterotopic pregnancy is rare but is seen commonly after artificial reproduction techniques. The presence of significant hemoperitoneum in the presence of an intrauterine pregnancy should raise the suspicion of heterotrophic pregnancy even if a mass has not been identified.

Ref: The role of ultrasonography in the diagnosis and management of early pregnancy complications

TOG 2015, Volume 17, 3

77. E

Desmopressin is preferable in intractable nocturia

Ref: (NICE CG 171, September, 2013: Urinary Incontinence in women: Management)

78. C

Duloxetine is the first line drug for SUI

Ref: (NICE CG 171, September, 2013: Urinary Incontinence in women: Management)

79. I

Bethanecol is a parasympathomimetic and can be used in urinary retention due to poor bladder contractility

80. B

In elderly frail ladies, oxybutynin should be avoided

Ref: (NICE CG 171, September, 2013: Urinary Incontinence in women: Management)

81. G

Ref: (NICE CG 171, September, 2013: Urinary Incontinence in women: Management)

82. D

Ref: (TOG: Management of vault prolapse: 2013; 15:167-170)

83. F

Ref: (TOG: Management of vault prolapse: 2013; 15:167-170)

84. F

Ref: (TOG: Management of vault prolapse: 2013; 15:167-170)

85. J

Ref: (RCOG GTG: 46: July 2015)

86. I

Ref: (RCOG GTG: 46: July 2015)

87. B

Ref: (RCOG GTG: 46: July 2015)

88. F

Girls over 13 years and less than 16 years can ask for termination and should be provided without parental consent if they meet Fraser competence *(NICE / FSRH evidence 2012)*

89. F

Girls over 13 years and less than 16 years can ask for termination and should be provided without parental consent if they meet Fraser competence *(NICE / FSRH evidence 2012)*

90. I

Paediatricians are trained in Level 3 child safeguarding to exclude child abuse / foul play and can also diagnose if it is a rash

91. C

There is a possibility of child abuse.

92. B

Ref: RCOG GTG 32: Management of Acute PID; BASHH UK national guideline for management of PID: June, 2011

93. A

Ofloxacin and Moxifloxacin should be avoided where there is a higher risk of Gonococci. Quinolone resistance is increasing

Ref: RCOG GTG 32: Management of Acute PID; BASHH UK national guideline for management of PID: June, 2011

94. C

Laparoscopy and drainage of pelvic abscess or ultrasound-guided drainage of abscess may be equally effective but there is no rational for routine salpingectomy or salpingo oophorectomy

Ref: RCOG GTG 32: Management of Acute PID; BASHH UK national guideline for management of PID: June, 2011

95. D

Intermenstrual bleeding and postcoital bleeding are more commonly associated with Chlamydial infection

96. D

Intermenstrual bleeding and postcoital bleeding are more commonly associated with Chlamydial infection

97. B

Clue cells are found in Bacterial vaginosis. They can be common during immunosuppression or following procedures like termination of pregnancy

98. F

Painful vaginal / vulval discharge or ulceration with lymphadenopathy can be Herpes simplex

99. I

Toxic shock syndrome can be caused following use of tampons. Staphylococcus aureus or Group A streptococcus are implicated.

100. H

Actinomycoces can be detected on smear in someone having a copper coil in situ. If symptomatic should be treated.

101. D

Cervical polyp can be incidentally found at time of cervical smear. One of the commonest associated symptoms is postcoital bleeding. It is most commonly benign and can be avulsed in the outpatients if it is present in the ectocervix.

102. A

Postmenopausal bleeding accounts for majority of the referral to the rapid access clinic. Only 10% women with postmenopausal bleeding have endometrial cancer or endometrial hyperplasia. Once the above is ruled out and if the vulva and vagina appears atrophic, a diagnosis of atrophic vaginitis can be made. The pattern of bleeding is usually small amount of spotting or staining of the underwear and has no pattern. It can be treated with short-term local oestrogen.

103. B

Cervix cancer can cause a number of symptoms. Sometimes it is detected after treatment for cervical intraepithelial neoplasia (CIN). Sometimes cervix cancer presents with abnormal vaginal bleeding, foul smelling discharge, or bleeding after intercourse. When advanced, cervix cancer can present by causing backache from a blockage of the tubes from the kidneys to the bladder (ureters).

104. J

This patient may have only pregnancy induced hypertension rather than pre-eclampsia. Whilst an isolated episode of + of protein may not be of concern but in view of raised blood pressure a baseline, urinary protein-creatinine ratio will help us quantify the proteinuria. Significant proteinuria is diagnosed if the urinary protein: creatinine ratio is greater than 30 mg/mmol or a 24-hour urine collection result shows greater than 300mg protein.

Ref: NICE Guidelines CG107 – Hypertension in pregnancy: diagnosis and management.

105. F

Assessing risk for gestational diabetes using risk factors is recommended in healthy population. At the booking appointment, the risk factors for gestational diabetes should be determined. For e.g. in this lady a BMI above 30kg/m^2 an OGTT to test for gestational diabetes at 24-28 weeks should be offered

Ref: NICE Guidelines CG62 – Antenatal care for uncomplicated pregnancies.

106. E

Other causes of itching and liver dysfunction should be excluded. Viral screen for Hepatitis A, B, C, Ebstein Barr and cytomegalovirus should be done

Ref: Obstetric Cholestasis Green-top Guideline No. 43

107. C

If the APH is associated with spontaneous or iatrogenic rupture of membranes, bleeding from a ruptured vasa praevia should be considered.

Ref: Antepartum Haemorrhage Green-top Guideline No. 63

108. E

If there is no maternal compromise in a patient with APH then a full history and examination should be performed to assess the amount and cause of bleeding. A speculum examination can be useful to identify cervical dilatation or visualize a lower genital cause for the APH. In a study of 389 women 21% had cervical ectropion on speculum examination

Ref: Antepartum Haemorrhage Green-top Guideline No. 63

109. H

Abnormal CTG is the most common consistent finding in uterine rupture and is present in 66-76% of these events

Ref: Birth after previous caesarean section Green-top Guideline No. 45

110. A

Cardiac disease was the most common indirect cause of maternal death in the MBRRACE report, 2015. The main cardiac cause of death is myocardial infarction, aortic dissection and cardiomyopathy.

Ref: Maternal collapse in pregnancy and the puerperium Green-top Guideline No. 56

111. H

Thromboembolism is the most common cause of direct death; hence clinical risk assessment and prophylaxis play an important role in improving maternal morbidity and mortality.

Ref: Maternal collapse in pregnancy and the pueperium Green-top Guideline No. 56

112. D

Amniotic fluid embolism presents as collapse during labour or delivery or within 30 minutes of delivery in the form of acute hypotension, respiratory distress and acute hypoxia.

Ref: Maternal collapse in pregnancy and the pueperium Green-top Guideline No. 56

113. E

Treponema pallidum causes syphilis and can be transmitted at any stage in pregnancy. The risk of transmission is dependent on the stage of maternal infection and duration of fetal exposure.

Ref: The management of sexually transmitted infections in pregnancy TOG 2012, Volume 14, 1

114. I

Gonorrhoea infection is associated with increased risk of preterm rupture of membranes, preterm birth and low birthweight. It also increases the risk of postpartum infection. Opthalmia neonatorum occurs in upto 50% of exposed babies.

Ref: The management of sexually transmitted infections in pregnancy TOG 2012, Volume 14, 1

115. J

Trichomonas vaginalis is associated with preterm birth and low birthweight. Little neonatal morbidity is associated with maternal T vaginalis.

Ref: The management of sexually transmitted infections in pregnancy TOG 2012, Volume 14, 1

116. J

Strawberry cervix with its characteristic vascular pattern is only present in 2% of the cases although this may be more visible at colposcopy

Ref: BASHH UK national guideline on management of trichomonas vaginalis 2007

117. H

The vaginal discharge for candida may be curdy having the appearance of small pieces of milk curd or cottage cheese like material within a pale gray or white discharge.

Ref: BASHH UK national guideline on management of vulvovaginal candidiasis 2007

118. A

The diagnosis of Herpes is confirmed by taking swabs from the infected lesions but treatment should not be withheld until the diagnosis is confirmed

Ref: BASHH UK national guideline on management of Genital herpes 2007

119. A

Pelvic pain that varies markedly over the menstrual cycle is likely to be attributable to a hormonally driven condition like endometriosis

Ref: The initial management of chronic pelvic pain Green-top Guideline No. 41

120. G

Rome III criteria for diagnosis of IBS

Ref: The initial management of chronic pelvic pain Green-top Guideline No. 41

121. F

Nerve entrapment in scar tissue, fascia or a narrow foramen may result in pain and dysfunction in the distribution of that nerve.

Ref: The initial management of chronic pelvic pain Green-top Guideline No. 41

122. F

Post pill amenorrhoea can last upto 6 months.

123. C

Once diagnosis of premature ovarian failure is confirmed, second line investigations such as Karyotyping and FMR-I premutation analysis are useful.

Ref: Diagnosis and management of premature ovarian failure
TOG 2011, Volume 13, 2

124. A

Serum prolactin should be routinely tested for secondary amenorrhoea. Since the mass is causing pressure effects on the optic chiasma, it is likely to be a macroprolactinoma and need referral to Endocrinologist and imaging.

125. G

Levonorgestrel-releasing intrauterine system (LNG-IUS) is the first line management

Ref: NICE Guidelines CG 44– Heavy menstrual bleeding: assessment and management

126. B

Danazol should not be routinely used for the treatment of HMB, but in cases of weight gain and hirsutism, can be used over COC pills.

Ref: NICE Guidelines CG 44– Heavy menstrual bleeding: assessment and management

127. E

Endometrial ablation should be considered in women who have a normal uterus and also those with small uterine fibroids (less than 3 cm in diameter). In women with HMB alone, with uterus no bigger than a 10-week pregnancy, endometrial ablation should be considered preferable to hysterectomy.

Ref: NICE Guidelines CG 44– Heavy menstrual bleeding: assessment and management

128. M

A laparoscopic approach should be considered in obese patient. Bilateral salpingo oophorectomy should be considered in view of her PMS.

Ref: NICE Guidelines CG 44– Heavy menstrual bleeding: assessment and management

129. L

Continuous or luteal phase (day 15-18) low dose SSRI is amongst the first line treatment of PMS

Ref: Management of premenstrual syndrome Green-top Guideline No. 48

130. A

When treating women with severe PMS, cognitive behavioural therapy should be considered routinely as a treatment option

Ref: Management of premenstrual syndrome Green-top Guideline No. 48

131. F

GNRH analogue therapy should be considered as second or third line therapy due to hypoestrogenic effect

Ref: Management of premenstrual syndrome Green-top Guideline No. 48

132. G

Benzathine benzylpenicillin G 2.4mu IM single dose for early syphilis in the first or second trimester.

Ref: The management of sexually transmitted infections in pregnancy TOG 2012, Volume 14, 1

133. A

Azithromycin 1g oral single dose is the first line for chlamydia

Ref: The management of sexually transmitted infections in pregnancy TOG 2012, Volume 14, 1

134. E

For recurrent herpes suppressive treatment is Acyclovir 400mg TDS in third trimester

Ref: The management of sexually transmitted infections in pregnancy TOG 2012, Volume 14, 1

135. E

Rudimentary horn can rupture if there is pregnancy in that horn.

Ref: Outflow tract disorders of the female genital tract TOG 2013, Volume 15, 1

136. A

Patients with Mayer Rokitansky Kuster Hauser syndrome present in their teenage years with primary amenorrhoea in the presence of normal secondary sexual characteristics. They have normal varies but absence of uterus and vagina means no menstruation

Ref: Outflow tract disorders of the female genital tract TOG 2013, Volume 15, 1

137. C

Transverse vaginal septum is much thicker hence it appears pink although bulging.

Ref: Outflow tract disorders of the female genital tract TOG 2013, Volume 15, 1

138. B

In contrast to vaginal septum, imperforate hymen reveals a bluish membrane with the dark blood trans illuminating.

Ref: Outflow tract disorders of the female genital tract TOG 2013, Volume 15, 1

139. H

Serotonin Norepinephrine Reuptake Inhibitor (SSNRI) will be treatment of choice as SSRIs paroxetine and fluoxetine should not be offered to women with breast cancer who are taking tamoxifen as it inhibits CYP2D6

Ref: Alternatives to HRT for the Management of the symptoms of the menopause

Scientific Impact Paper No: 6

140. G

The selective serotonin re-uptake inhibitor (SSRI) antidepressants paroxetine [14] and fluoxetine [14] may be offered to women with breast cancer for relieving menopausal symptoms, particularly hot flushes, but not to those taking tamoxifen.

Ref: Alternatives to HRT for the Management of the symptoms of the menopause

Scientific Impact Paper No: 6

141. E

Women with vaginal dryness can use moisturisers and lubricants such as Replens.

Ref: Alternatives to HRT for the Management of the symptoms of the menopause

cientific Impact Paper No: 6

142. D

FFP at a dose of 12–15 ml/kg should be administered for every 6 units of red cells during major obstetric haemorrhage.

Ref: Blood transfusion in Obstetrics

Green-top Guideline No. 47

143. C

Cryoprecipitate at a standard dose of two 5-unit pools should be administered early in major obstetric haemorrhage. Subsequent cryoprecipitate transfusion should be guided by fibrinogen results, aiming to keep levels above 1.5 g/l.

Ref: Blood transfusion in Obstetrics

Green-top Guideline No. 47

144. H

A platelet transfusion trigger of 75 x 109/l is recommended to provide a margin of safety.

Ref: Blood transfusion in Obstetrics
Green-top Guideline No. 47

145. C

Clinicians should perform clinical examination in all women suspected of endometriosis, although vaginal examination may be inappropriate for adolescents and/or women without previous sexual intercourse. In such cases, rectal examination can be helpful for the diagnosis of endometriosis.

146. J

Most likely chlamydia infection hence ideal site for swab is endocervical and rectal

147. F

Every patient presenting with urinary incontinence should be examined for prolapse and the ideal position for assessment of vaginal prolapse is Sims position

148. I

Where the torn internal anal sphincter (IAS) can be identified, it is advisable to repair this separately with interrupted or mattress sutures without any attempt to overlap the IAS. A monofilament suture such as 3-0 PDS should be used.

149. A

Where the torn internal anal sphincter (IAS) can be identified, it is advisable to repair this separately with interrupted or mattress sutures without any attempt to overlap the IAS. A monofilament suture such as 3-0 PDS should be used. 3-0 polyglactin should be used to repair the anorectal mucosa as it may cause less irritation and discomfort.

Ref: The management of Third- and Fourth-degree Perineal tear.
Green-top Guideline No. 29

150. I

For partial thickness (all 3a and some 3b) tears, an end-to-end technique should be used. When repair of the EAS and/or IAS muscle is being performed, either monofilament sutures such as 3-0 PDS or modern braided sutures such as 2-0 polyglactin can be used with equivalent outcomes.

Ref: The management of Third- and Fourth-degree Perineal tears Green-top Guideline No. 29

151. A

Pregnancy, raised BMI and long haul flights are all risk factors for venous thromboembolism. With the tachycardia and hypoxia, pulmonary embolism should be high on the list of differential diagnosis

152. G

Bilateral pedal oedema, hepatomegaly makes Heart failure the likely diagnosis. Fluid shift and advancing pregnancy may make symptoms worse. Raised blood pressure is a risk factor

153. D

Anaemia is common in twin gestations and can present as dizziness, tiredness and headaches. Iron supplementation is recommended in multiple gestations

154. E

With the gestational diabetes, there is a risk of polyhydramnios, which is likely to pose some difficulties palpating fetal parts. Women with Polyhydramnios are likely to measure large for gestational age and present with shortness of breath.

155. J

This woman has fever, and a productive cough together with the chest symptoms. In pregnancy chest infections can present as pain in the upper abdomen

156. H

All her vital signs are normal apart from mild tachycardia. After having a scan showing an anomaly she is likely to be anxious

157. G

Appendicitis is the most common acute abdominal condition in pregnancy. Appendicitis presents usually with pain around the umbilicus and later at the right lower quadrant, nausea, vomiting and anorexia. Be aware that in pregnancy patients with appendicitis may present with non-classic symptoms. The pain may be in the right upper quadrant or they may even present with heartburn

TOG 2015; VOL 17, 2

158. I

This colicky nature and vomiting makes gastroenteritis the likely diagnosis. There is usually a history of people with whom she had been in contact having the same symptoms. They can be associated with diarrhoea and usually self-limiting.

159. A

Placental abruption can be associated with pre eclampsia and the retroplacental clot causes the severe abdominal pain or the irritable uterus. In severe cases it leads to fetal demise and gives the classical "woody hard" feeling on palpating the abdomen. Note the raised blood pressure of this woman

160. C

Musculoskeletal pain is common in pregnancy and usually worse on movements. Relaxin and progesterone in pregnancy causes relaxation of joints. This together with the stretching of muscles, pressure from the enlarging gravid uterus contributes to the musculoskeletal symptoms of pregnancy. The small cyst is unlikely to be the cause of the pain.

161. J

Fibroid is the most likely cause of pain in this case. Most fibroids are asymptomatic in pregnancy but they can cause severe pain when they undergo red degeneration. One of the theories behind the pain is the rapid growth of the fibroid that can occur in pregnancy resulting in it outgrowing its blood supply. Management is with analgesia and hydration.

162. J

Nulliparous women with uncomplicated pregnancies should be offered a membrane sweep at 40 and 41 weeks. They should be offered Induction of labour between 41 and 42 weeks

Ref: NICE (CG 70): Inducing labour

163. A

With a Bishops Score of 5 it is likely that ARM can be done. The first step for this woman is to do an ARM and await spontaneous contractions. Syntocinon may be used to augment labour but one should be aware of the risk associated with it and the woman should be informed. It is recommended that syntocinon be used in women with a caesarean scar only after discussion with a consultant or senior obstetrician. Although Prostaglandin can be given, however, in view of previous caesarean section and the risk of uterine rupture, it would be at the discretion of a Senior Obstetrician.

Ref: NICE (CG 70): Inducing labour

164. B

Prolonged rupture of membranes is a risk for infection. As she is term, labour should be augmented. As she is not contracting, Syntocinon is the suitable agent to use. The risk associated with syntocinon use (including scar rupture) should be explained and this should be discussed with a senior obstetrician.

Ref: NICE (CG 70): Inducing labour

165. H

Although it seems she has a Bishops score of 7 and hence ARM can be done, this baby is growth restricted and compromised and unlikely to cope with the labour. Induction of labour is not recommended and the baby will need delivery by caesarean section

Ref: NICE (CG 70): Inducing labour

166. I

This woman will not need any intervention at this stage and it is likely she will go into spontaneous labour. If not delivered she should be offered membrane sweep at 41 weeks and induction of labour between 41 and 42 weeks

Ref: NICE (CG 70): Inducing labour

167. E

At this gestation, misoprostol at a lower dose is likely to be more effective than prostaglandins. The woman should be informed that both are not without risk. Although not licensed in the UK for this purpose, it has been endorsed by NICE for induction following IUD in women with a previous caesarean section

Ref: NICE (CG 70): Inducing labour

168. E

Delay in first stage of labour is diagnosed when there is less than 2cm cervical dilatation in 4hrs. Dysfunctional uterine contractions are a common cause of delay in first stage and syntocinon in incremental dose till there are 4-5 regular contractions every 10 minutes is recommended.

Ref: NICE (CG 190): Intrapartum care

169. A

This is cord presentation. As the membrane is intact she does not need urgent, delivery and can be delivered by a grade 2 caesarean section

Ref: NICE (CG 190): Intrapartum care

170. B

As opposed to the above question, this is cord prolapse and should be delivered urgently. If this is diagnosed at second stage, forceps if suitable can expedite delivery.

Ref: NICE (CG 190): Intrapartum care

171. E

Although grand multiparous women are likely to deliver without any intervention, it is expected that there should be at least 2cm of cervical dilatation every 4 hours. Syntocinon use in grandmultiparous women poses a risk of uterine rupture and in most cases all that is required will be to rupture the membranes and adequate contractions and delivery will follow

Ref: NICE (CG 190): Intrapartum care

172. J

In this case the cervix is unlikely to be favourable at this stage of pregnancy. Further prostaglandin is not appropriate and there is no reason why the process should not be paused and restarted after a period of rest .A discussion should take place with the woman regarding giving a period of rest about 48hrs and repeating the process. Such women should stay in hospital and the baby monitored regularly

Ref: NICE (CG 190): Intrapartum care

173. A

This is likely to be deep transverse arrest. With a failed progress and signs of obstruction, the most appropriate management will be by caesarean section. Caesarean section for this reason does not need to be done as a grade 1

Ref: NICE (CG 190): Intrapartum care

174. K

Although having 4 contractions every 10min, they are irregular. For a primiparous woman, she will need syntocinon infusion to regularise the contractions and help with rotation of the fetal head. It is important to assess the women to exclude signs of obstruction before commencing syntocinon at the second stage

Ref: NICE (CG 190): Intrapartum care

175. D

This woman has been pushing for the last 90minute. Although birth should be expected within 2 hours, the CTG is abnormal and the baby needs to be delivered. A non-rotational forceps is the most appropriate means of delivery in this case. A ventouse delivery is more likely to fail in view of the caput. Having said that, the choice of the instrument will also depend on the skills and preference of the operator

Ref: NICE (CG 190): Intrapartum care

176. H

This woman does not need intervention now. Delivery is expected within 3 hours in first deliveries and in the absence of maternal or fetal compromise, intervention is only required after 2 hours of pushing without delivery

Ref: NICE (CG 190): Intrapartum care

177. D

In face presentation, vaginal delivery is possible if presenting in mento anterior position as opposed to mento posterior position. As she has been pushing effectively for 1 hour, intervention is required unless delivery is eminent. The ventouse cup cannot be used on a face presentation.

Ref: NICE (CG 190): Intrapartum care

178. B

The slow progress in the later stages of the first stage may indicate that the labour is getting obstructed. The examination findings are not suitable for an operative vaginal delivery and should be delivered by caesarean section especially with a caesarean section scar. Syntocinon infusion or further wait is not appropriate and the caesarean section need not be grade 1.

RCOG GTG: 26: Operative vaginal delivery

179. J

With an abnormal CTG, the baby needs to deliver. Being preterm it is likely that the fetal head could be easily rotated and delivery expedited straight away with forceps. Caution should be taken when performing manual rotation, as the fetal head is likely to be soft. Caesarean section could be an option but delivery is more likely to be quicker and safer vaginally. Ventouse cup should not be used for deliveries below 34 weeks, as its safety is uncertain.

Ref: NICE (CG 190): Intrapartum care

180. L

The CTG is abnormal showing features that are likely to lead to acidosis if no intervention is taken. Being multiparous and with the rapid progress she is likely to progress rapidly again in the second stage and either deliver spontaneously or easily with an operative delivery. Although an FBS is not contraindicated with meconium, you should be thinking of delivery of the baby at this stage. With the risk of fetal acidosis one should be thinking about caeasarean section if vaginal deliver (operative is proving difficult). In this scenario the reasonable option will be L

Ref: NICE (CG 190): Intrapartum care

181. D

Operative vaginal delivery can be performed in most of cord prolapse at second stage especially if vaginal examination findings predict a quick, easy and safe operative vaginal delivery. Both forceps and the vacuum extractor can be used but the forceps is less likely to impinge on the prolapsed cord and more likely to achieve delivery quicker

RCOG GTG 50: Umbilical Cord Prolapse

182. C

This is common and affects about 80-85% of women after birth. This is considered as normal and usually due to hormonal readjustments where women go through a brief period of feeling low in the first week after delivery. Although feeling low they are able to cope with normal activities and do not get symptoms of depression. Some women may be irritable during this period.

NICE CG: 192: Antenatal and Postnatal Mental Health: Clinical Management and Service Guidance

183. D

Endometritis is the most likely diagnosis. It is unlikely to be a wound infection with the wound looking clean. A speculum examination may reveal offensive lochia but this was declined due to pain. This need prompt treatment as can progress to septicaemia if untreated.

RCOG GTG 64B: Sepsis following pregnancy

184. A

This woman has showing signs and symptoms of Psychosis including grandiose delusions. This is a psychiatric emergency and will need specialist attention, as there can be significant danger to the mother baby and people around her. Presentation is usually acute onset. Risk factors include a past history or family history of psychiatric illness eg. Bipolar disorder

NICE CG: 192: Antenatal and Postnatal Mental Health: Clinical Management and Service Guidance

185. F

Mastitis is inflammation of breast tissue that can results from stasis of milk from blocked ducts, an infection or a combination of the two. If untreated this can lead to an abscess, which usually presents as a fluctuant area or lump on the breast. A fluctuant area or lump is not mentioned in this question.

RCOG GTG 64B: Sepsis following pregnancy

186. E

The patients' vital signs suggest that she has got sepsis. Sepsis is an important cause of maternal death in the puerperium with genital tract being the commonest source. The tachycardia, hypotension and fever (sometimes hypothermia) should raise a strong suspicion of sepsis and trigger immediate investigations and prompt management. These include blood cultures, broad-spectrum antibiotic within 1 hour of the suspicion as recommended by the SSCB, serum lactate and relevant imaging

RCOG GTG 64B: Sepsis following pregnancy

187. K

Post-natal depression affects about 10-15%. This usually begins some weeks or months after birth and can last for about a year. In addition to the symptoms of depression, they find it difficult to cope with looking after their baby concentrate and some may need medications. *NICE CG: 192: Antenatal and Postnatal Mental Health: Clinical Management and Service Guidance*

188. H

Striae gravidarum is very common in pregnancy. It is non itchy and the linear purple changes results from rupture of elastic fibres of the skin. More common with overstretching and affects usually abdomen and buttocks

189. C

Obstetrics cholestasis usually presents as intense itch worse at night and involves the hands and feet including the palms and sole. Typically there are no rashes

190. E

Polymorphic eruption of pregnancy typically spares the periumbilical area

191. I

The blisters and bullous lesions are typical of pemphigoid. It is also common in women with autoimmune conditions such as Graves's disease.

192. A

Atopic eruption usually presents as papular and nodular excoriated lesions on the face, trunk and chest. A family history of atopy is a risk

193. F

Chicken pox presents as maculopapular rash later developing to vesicles spreading usually from the trunk to the extremities. Fever is a common feature and the scalp is involved

(188-193): TOG, Vol 15, 4, Oct 2013, skin eruptions in pregnancy

194. A
Previous history of DVT

195. J
Varicosities alone is not an indication for thromboprophylaxis

196. I
LMWH is unsuitable for patients with mechanical valves. They are likely to be on long-term warfarin, which may have been converted to LMWH during pregnancy.
Their anticoagulant should be converted back to warfarin after delivery. Warfarin is also safe to use in breastfeeding women.

197. J
Elective caesarean section with no other risk factors

198. B
Readmission is an indication

199. B
She has 2 risk factors: Intrauterine fetal death and smoking

200. A
Thromboprophylaxis should be delayed for at least four hours after removal epidural catheter or regional anaesthesia to reduce the risk of haematoma.

201. G
The catheter should be removed after 4 hours

Ref: For questions 194-201, see RCOG Green-top Guidelines No 37A. Thrombosis and Embolism during pregnancy and puerperium, reducing the Risk

SINGLE BEST ANSWERS (SBAs)

1. D

Evidence suggests the use of hyaluronic acid derivatives, PEG derivatives and solid barrier agents are the best anti adhesive agents for both laparoscopic and hysteroscopic surgery. Little evidence for Icodextrin (Adept) as an anti adhesive agent.

Ref: The Use of Adhesion Prevention agents in Obstetrics & Gynaecology Scientific Impact Paper: 39

2. B

The underlying physiological process causing malignant ascites is often multifactorial and may be due to obstruction of lymphatic drainage preventing absorption of intra-abdominal fluid and protein, hypoproteinaemia and occasionally portal hypertension secondary to hepatic cancer. Non-malignant ascites is due to over production of fluid. The lymphatic flow is increased to 200mls/hr.

Ref: Management of Ascitis in Ovarian Cancer Patients Scientific Impact Paper: 45

3. C

Roux- n-Y gastric bypass is both a malabsorptive and restrictive type of bariatric surgery. All other procedures mentioned in the question are restrictive type of surgery.

Ref: The role of Bariatric Surgery in Improving Reproductive Health Scientific Impact Paper: 17

4. A

The only factor that is proven to be improved is the miscarriage rate as pre-pregnancy obesity and gestational weight gain is associated with increased risk of miscarriage.

Ref: The role of Bariatric Surgery in Improving Reproductive Health Scientific Impact Paper: 17

5. C

The risk of endometrioid endometrial cancer is highest in obsese woman due to increased oestrogen production.

Ref: Endometrial Cancer in Obese Women
Scientific Impact Paper: 32

6. C

Its FIGO Stage 1B endometrial cancer. The ideal treatment is surgery. In a large BMI patient, it is recommended to perform laparoscopic hysterectomy + BSO as it reduces length of stay in the hospital, wound infection rate, recovery time and superior quality of life styles.

Ref: Endometrial Cancer in Obese Women
Scientific Impact Paper: 32

7. D

Enhanced recovery pathway entails clear fluid up to 2 hours prior to surgery, avoiding long acting sedative, administration of antibiotic prior to incision and decreasing the volume of intravenous fluid with early feeding.

Ref: Enhanced Recovery in Gynaecology
Scientific Impact Paper: 36

8. B

Ref: Fertility-sparing Treatments in Gynaecological Cancers
Scientific Impact Paper: 35

9. A

Radical vaginal trachelectomy is usually restricted to tumour size <2cm as the recurrence rate is higher in bigger tumour sizes.

Ref: Fertility-sparing Treatments in Gynaecological Cancers
Scientific Impact Paper: 35

10. A

Ablation technique is only suitable if the whole transformation zone is visible and there is no major discrepancy between the cytology and histology. Although there is a difference in the histological and colposcopic assessment but both grades the lesion as high grade.

Ref: NHS Cervical Screening Programme (NHSCSP) Publication No. 20

11. E

The depth of excision should be at least 7mm (<10mm) in transformation zone (TZ) type 1. In type 2 TZ, this should be 10 – 15mm and in type 3 TZ, this should be 15 – 25mm.
Ref: NHS Cervical Screening Programme (NHSCSP) Publication No. 20

12. B

A pregnant woman should have colposcopy in late first trimester or early 2nd trimester for an abnormal cytology.
Ref: NHS Cervical Screening Programme (NHSCSP) Publication No. 20

13. B

Systemic chemotherapy is safe in the 2nd trimester of pregnancy but contraindicated in the 1st trimester of pregnancy. Radiotherapy is contraindicated until delivery. Tamoxifen is contraindicated in pregnancy.
Ref: Pregnancy and Breast Cancer
Green-top Guideline No. 12

14. C

Echocardiography should be performed during pregnancy in women at risk to detect cardiomyopathy through resting left ventricular ejection fraction or echocardiographic fractional shortening.
Ref: Pregnancy and Breast Cancer
Green-top Guideline No. 12

15. C

Ref: Management of Endometrial Hyperplasia
Green-top Guideline No. 67

16. E

The gold standard investigation to rule out endometrial pathology is hysteroscopy and endometrial biopsy.
Ref: Management of Endometrial Hyperplasia
Green-top Guideline No. 67

17. E

Miniature hysteroscopes – 2.7mm with a 3 – 3.5mm sheath is ideal for outpatient hysteroscopy as it reduces the discomfort to the women.
Ref: Best Practice in Outpatient Hysteroscopy
Green-top Guideline No. 59

18. A

Normal saline is the distention medium to be used if bipolar diathermy is used for electrosurgery and glycine is needed for monopolar surgery. However, evidence suggests that the rate of vasovagal episodes is reduced with normal saline.
Ref: Best Practice in Outpatient Hysteroscopy
Green-top Guideline No. 59

19. E

The veress needle and the primary trocar should be inserted at 90° to the skin. This is to prevent tenting and increasing the distance to be traversed by the needle or the trocar.
Ref: Preventing Entry Related Gynaecological Laparoscopic Injuries
Green-top Guideline No. 49

20. B

The rate of adhesions following a midline laparotomy is 50% and is 23% after a low transverse incision. The preferred alternate entry method should be Palmer's point entry unless there is history of splenic surgery. Hasson open entry technique can also be used.
Ref: Preventing Entry Related Gynaecological Laparoscopic Injuries
Green-top Guideline No. 49

21. D

The risk of vascular injury is highest in very thin woman as the aorta only lies 2.5cm away from the umbilicus.
Ref: Preventing Entry Related Gynaecological Laparoscopic Injuries
Green-top Guideline No. 49

22. C

Patient specific concern should be checked prior to starting surgery as per the WHO Surgical checklist

Ref: WHO surgical checklist

http://www.nrls.npsa.nhs.uk/resources/clinical-specialty/surgery/?entryid45=59860

23. A

The ASA Grade is confirmed prior to surgery after anesthetising the patient. The rest of the checks are performed prior to induction of anaesthesia.

Ref: WHO surgical checklist

http://www.nrls.npsa.nhs.uk/resources/clinical-specialty/surgery/?entryid45=59860

24. C

The risk of ovarian malignancy increases by threefold after the age of 50.

Ref: Management of Suspected Ovarian Masses in Premenopausal Women

Green-top Guideline No. 62

25. C

Chemical peritonitis is a rare complication of surgery especially laparoscopic surgery for dermoid cyst.

Ref: Management of Suspected Ovarian Masses in Premenopausal Women

Green-top Guideline No. 62

26. D

The failure rate of hysteroscopic sterilization is uncommon.

Ref: Female Sterilization

RCOG Consent Advice No.3

27. D

The survival rate after chemotherapy in women with epithelial ovarian cancer is reasonably high.

Ref: The Distal Fallopian Tube as the Origin of Non-Uterine Pelvic High-Grade Serous Carcinomas

Scientific Impact Paper No. 44

28. B

In patients with suspected Stage 1 Ovarian Cancer (confined to the ovary), a staging surgery with retroperitoneal lymph node assessment should be performed. Block dissection of the lymph nodes from the pelvic sidewalls upto the level of the renal vein should not be done if the disease is confined to the ovaries.

Ref: NICE Guidelines CG122 – Ovarian Cancer: recognition and initial management

29. E

Ref: NICE Guidelines CG122 – Ovarian Cancer: recognition and initial management

30. C

6 doses of carboplatin are used for adjuvant chemotherapy. The 2nd line drug would be paclitaxel.

Ref: NICE Guidelines CG122 – Ovarian Cancer: recognition and initial management

31. B

Ref: FIGO Staging of Endometrial Cancer
http://emedicine.medscape.com/article/2006791-overview

32. D

Ref: FIGO Staging in Vulval and Endometrial Cancer
TOG 2010, Volume 2012, 4

33. B

Sentinel lymph node biopsy has been introduced to reduce morbidity. Radical inguinal lymphadenectomy is associated with significant morbidity. However, lymph node involvement is the most important prognostic factor. Therefore, it is important for biopsy. In the past, systematic inguinofemoral node dissection was performed.

Ref: FIGO Staging in Vulval and Endometrial Cancer
TOG 2010, Volume 2012, 4

34. D

The wound dehiscence risk is highest with midline incision. However it is least hemorrhagic and the nerve damage is also more with the lower transverse incision. It is slow to enter the abdomen and obviously it is not cosmetically best for the patient.

Ref: Abdominal Incisions and Sutures in Obstetrics and Gynaecology
TOG 2014, Volume 16, 1

35. C

Mersilene suture is a braided suture with high tensile strength and low tissue reaction. It is a non- absorbable suture.

Ref: Abdominal Incisions and Sutures in Obstetrics and Gynaecology
TOG 2014, Volume 16, 1

36. E

100% silicon catheter should be used to reduce infection rate.

Ref: Catheter use in gynaecological practice
TOG 2014, Volume 16, 3

37. E

Suprapubic catheterisation is contraindicated if the patient is on anticoagulation therapy and if a pelvic mass is present.

Ref: Catheter use in gynaecological practice
TOG 2014, Volume 16, 3

38. A

Ref: Urinary tract injuries in laparoscopic gynaecological surgery; prevention, recognition and management
TOG 2014, Volume 16, 1

39. A

The type of ureteric repair depends on the site and type of injury.

Ref: Urinary tract injuries in laparoscopic gynaecological surgery; prevention, recognition and management
TOG 2014, Volume 16, 1

40. E

In Retrograde cystography, the contrast fills the bladder gradually and a series of X ray is performed. Healing is confirmed by the absence of leakage. Micturating cystourethogram is performed where a fistula is suspected.

Ref: Urinary tract injuries in laparoscopic gynaecological surgery; prevention, recognition and management
TOG 2014, Volume 16, 1

41. C

Genitofemoral nerve is susceptible to injury during pelvic sidewall surgery such as external iliac lymph node dissection. As this nerve bifurcates into a genital and femoral branch. Damage to this nerve would cause parasthesia over mons pubis, labia majoram and femoral triangle.
Ref: Nerve Injuries associated with gynaecological surgeries
TOG 2014, Volume 16, 1

42. C

Hydrodilatation is a safer method of dilatation than mechanical dilatation. With a 30° hysteroscope, the cervical os should be at 6'o clock position in an anteverted uterus with the light cable down and at 12'o clock position with a retroverted uterus with the light cable vertically up. If the light cable is held down irrespective of the version of the uterus, then the cervical os should always be at 6'o clock position. In a 0° hysteroscope, the cervical canal should be centrally placed.
Ref: Failed hysteroscopies and further management strategies
TOG 2016, Volume 18, 1

43. C

The validity of consent is based on 3 factors – capacity, information and free will. Refusing surgery does not show lack of capacity. Being in pain or hemodynamic unstable if the patient is able to understand the information does no cause lack of capacity. However, being influenced by a family member or friend makes the refusal invalid and the Court of Protection can be approached if the procedure is deemed necessary for the life of the patient.
Ref: Consent in Clinical Practice
TOG 2015, Volume 17, 4

44. A

Ref: Surgical Procedures and Postoperative Care
StratOG Core Module

45. B

Testosterone levels are high in Leydig Cell Tumour as these are the cells in the ovary, which secretes excess testosterone.
Ref: Gynaecological Oncology
StratOG Core Module

46. D

The gynaecology risk trigger is blood loss on ≥ 500mls during gynaecological surgery.
Ref: Improving Patient Safety: Risk Management for Maternity and Gynaecology
RCOG Clinical Governance Advice No. 2

47. E

A consultant should lead the gynaecology risk team with special interest in gynaecology risk management. The team should have the lead gynaecology nurse, theatre practitioner, ultrasonographer and the service manager. However, the MDT coordinator need not be a part of this team.
Ref: Improving Patient Safety: Risk Management for Maternity and Gynaecology
RCOG Clinical Governance Advice No. 2

48. A

The audit cycle has steps as described.
Ref: Understanding Audit
RCOG Clinical Governance Advice No. 2

49. B

Statistical Analysis
Ref: StratOG Module – The Obstetrician & Gynaecologist as a Teacher and Researcher

50. C

Statistical Analysis

Ref: StratOG Module – The Obstetrician & Gynaecologist as a Teacher and Researcher

51. E

Statistical Analysis

Ref: StratOG Module – The Obstetrician & Gynaecologist as a Teacher and Researcher

52. C

Statistical Analysis

Ref: StratOG Module – The Obstetrician & Gynaecologist as a Teacher and Researcher

53. E

High FSH, low AMH and antral follicle count suggests she is almost in premature menopause.

54. A

There is no increased risk of ovarian or breast cancer and no increased surveillance is necessary. In amenorrhoea in PCOS, gestogens should be used every 3-4 months to induce bleed. If endometrium is thickened, endometrial biopsy and preferably hysteroscopy to exclude hyperplasia.

(Ref: (NICE CG33: Long term consequences of Polycystic Ovary Syndrome)

55. D

Clomiphene is not advised beyond 6 months. In clomiphene resistance, either clomiphene + metformin or gonadotrophins or ovarian drilling are advised.

Ref: (NICE CG156: Fertility Problems: Assessment and Treatment)

56. C

She has hypothalamic (WHO Type 1) anovulation. Therefore, either pulsatile GnRH or gonadotrophins are effective but gonadotrophins are generally used because of ease of administration.

Ref: (NICE CG156: Fertility Problems: Assessment and Treatment)

57. C

Hypothalamo - Pituitary Type 1 ovulatory disorder can be treated with either Pulsatile GnRH or Gonadotrophins: Sheehan's syndrome

Ref: (NICE CG156: Fertility Problems: Assessment and Treatment)

58. E

In unexplained subfertility, no indication to give Clomiphene and IUI is indicated only in few definitive indications

Ref: (NICE CG156: Fertility Problems: Assessment and Treatment)

59. E

Surgical treatment for mild or moderate endometriosis is preferred but if it does not help then IVF is the next step. IUI is not an option.

Ref: (NICE CG156: Fertility Problems: Assessment and Treatment)

60. B

Prolactin and testosterone are relevant in oligomenorrhoea. Because on anovulation, FSH is more relevant than Thyroid function. With such irregular cycles day 21 progesterone is less likely to be representative and the cycles are most likely anovulatory.

61. D

Hysterosalpingogram is the first choice

Ref: (NICE CG156: Fertility Problems: Assessment and Treatment)

62. C

Since she has a history of possible PID and also ectopic pregnancy, Laparoscopy and treatment if feasible is the preferred method

Ref: (NICE CG156: Fertility Problems: Assessment and Treatment)

63. A

He has hypogonadotrophic hypogonadism.

64. E

Antisperm antibodies are not part of the routine investigations and steroids have no role.

Ref: (NICE CG156: Fertility Problems: Assessment and Treatment)

65. D

Lutcal phase support with progesterone is advised in IVF

Ref: (NICE CG156: Fertility Problems: Assessment and Treatment)

66. C

In WHO Type I ovulatory disorder, Gonadotrophin therapy must include HCG/LH

Ref: (NICE CG156: Fertility Problems: Assessment and Treatment)

67. C

Ref: (NICE CG 154: Ectopic pregnancy and miscarriage: Diagnosis and initial management)

68. C

Ref: (NICE CG 154: Ectopic pregnancy and miscarriage: Diagnosis and initial management)

69. E

First line of management is expectant management

Ref: (NICE CG 154: Ectopic pregnancy and miscarriage: Diagnosis and initial management)

70. C

Below 6 weeks if patient does not have any pain, repeat urine pregnancy test in 1 week before considering ultrasound scan

Ref: (NICE CG 154: Ectopic pregnancy and miscarriage: Diagnosis and initial management)

71. E

Pregnancy of uncertain viability should have repeat ultrasound scan – if transvaginal: in 1 week, if transabdominal: in 2 weeks

Ref: (NICE CG 154: Ectopic pregnancy and miscarriage: Diagnosis and initial management)

72. E

In PUL with HCG that has plateaued, should be reviewed by Senior Gynaecologist

Ref: (NICE CG 154: Ectopic pregnancy and miscarriage: Diagnosis and initial management)

73. D

Mifepristone is not recommended for early miscarriage. It is recommended for termination of pregnancy

Ref: (NICE CG 154: Ectopic pregnancy and miscarriage: Diagnosis and initial management)

74. B

Methotrexate can only be given if patient has pain that is not significant, HCG less than 5000 and adnexal mass less than 35 mm although the patient should be counselled that the risk of treatment failure is high at HCG levels greater than 3500.

Ref: (NICE CG 154: Ectopic pregnancy and miscarriage: Diagnosis and initial management)

75. D

Ref: (NICE CG 154: Ectopic pregnancy and miscarriage: Diagnosis and initial management)

76. C

Although smoking and caffeine are considered a risk factor, there is insufficient evidence. Advanced maternal age of 35 and above and paternal age of 40 and above are risk factors

Ref: (RCOG GTG 17: The Investigation and Treatment of Couples with Recurrent first trimester and Second trimester miscarriage)

77. D

Ref: (RCOG GTG 17: The Investigation and Treatment of Couples with Recurrent first trimester and Second trimester miscarriage)

78. D

Parental karyotyping should be performed only where there is unbalanced structural chromosomal abnormality on testing the products of conception.

Women with 2nd trimester miscarriage should be tested for hereditary thrombophilias

Ref: (RCOG GTG 17: The Investigation and Treatment of Couples with Recurrent first trimester and Second trimester miscarriage)

79. B

She has reduced bladder capacity of 380ml (normal: 450-500ml). She has detrusor activity during filling phase and with tapwater. Her first desire to void is at 140ml (normal: 150-200 ml). She has some stress incontinence (leaks little urine on repeated coughing) but the predominant diagnosis is Detrusor overactivity. She also has some voiding difficulty (residual volume >50ml)

80. B

Painful Bladder syndrome is characterized by pain during filling phase along with other symptoms like frequency, nocturia in the absence of proven UTI.
Ref: (TOG: 2007: Vol.9, 1)

81. B

Petechial haemorrhages are found in Interstitial cystitis. Sensory urgency is considered the milder end of the spectrum of Painful bladder syndrome, while Interstitial cystitis is the extreme end.
Ref: (TOG: 2007: Vol.9, 1)

82. E

At the first visit, pelvic floor muscle tone should be assessed before pelvic floor muscle training
Ref: (NICE CG 171: Urinary Incontinence in women)

83. B

Test urine in all women presenting to urogynaecology clinic but do not treat if they are asymptomatic even if leucocytes and nitrites are positive. Instead, send mid stream urine for culture and sensitivity and treat if positive. However, treat at the initial visit if symptomatic and dipstick is positive for both leucocytes and nitrites.
Ref: (NICE CG 171: Urinary Incontinence in women)

84. B

Both bladder scans and catheterization post void are preferred methods to assess residual urine volume in voiding difficulties but bladder scan should be used first because of acceptability and less adverse effects.
Ref: (NICE CG 171: Urinary Incontinence in women)

85. E

Ref: (NICE CG 171: Urinary Incontinence in women)

86. A

In a small group of patients where detailed history and clinical examination suggests pure stress urinary incontinence, will not need urodynamics prior to surgery.

Ref: (NICE CG 171: Urinary Incontinence in women)

87. C

Suprapubic catheters are preferred over long-term urethral catheters because of less infection, bypassing,

Ref: (NICE CG 171: Urinary Incontinence in women)

88. B

Oxybutinin, Tolteradine and Darifenacin are first line drugs for Overactive bladder syndrome. However, Oxybutinin is not well tolerated by elderly frail ladies.

Ref: (NICE CG 171: Urinary Incontinence in women

89. B

If oxybutynin is effective but not tolerated orally, transdermal oxybutynin is an option.

Ref: (NICE CG 171: Urinary Incontinence in women)

90. B

91. E

92. A

Young adults with a history of non-compliance with taking pills, long-term injectable contraception is acceptable and advisable. IUCD is permissible but less commonly prescribed because of the risk of STI and acceptability.

Ref: (NICE: CG30: Long acting reversible contraception)

93. E

18 year old with postcoital bleeding: Chlamydia needs to be excluded

94. A

Transvaginal ultrasound is less invasive than laparoscopy and can reveal hydrosalpinx, tuboovarian mass and exclude other differentials eg. Ovarian cysts or endometrioma.

Ref: (RCOG GTG 32: PID; BASHH: UK National guideline for management of PID)

95. C

In sexual assault where vaginal penetration is suspected, the following swabs should be taken: vulval, perineal, vaginal: high and low, speculum, lubricant, pubic hair, endocervical

Ref: (Oxford Handbook of Obstetrics & Gynaecology)

96. C

STI indicative of child sexual abuse are: Gonorrhoea (over 1 year), Syphilis and HIV (if congenital infection excluded), Chlamydia (over 3 years). Herpes simplex can be non-sexually transmitted as well

Ref: (Oxford Handbook of Obstetrics & Gynaecology)

97. B

VTE risks: Background risk: 5:100,000; 2nd Generation COC pills: 10-15:100,000; 3rd Generation COC pills: 25:100,000; Pregnancy: 60:100,000

Ref: (Oxford Handbook of Obstetrics & Gynaecology)

98. D

While breast-feeding progesterone only pill would be preferred over COC pill. This can be affected by hepatic enzyme affecting drugs but not by antibiotics (unlike COC pills)

99. B

Women at higher risk of regret for taking the decision to adopt permanent method of sterilization: less than 30 years (current RCOG recommendation is to avoid), who do not have children, who decide during pregnancy, who have had a recent relationship loss

100. D

Mechanism of action is fibrosis; it is made of metal, and not recommended less than 30 years of age *(RCOG)*

101. B

Levonelle is effective upto 72 hours (3 days), Ella one and Copper IUCD upto 120 hours (5 days) but Copper IUCD is the most effective. The Failure rate is less than 1%

102. E

She needs sequential preparation as LMP not > 12 months

Ref: NICE Guidelines NG23 –Menopause: Diagnosis and management

103. D

Diagnosis of premature ovarian failure is if elevated FSH levels on 2 blood samples taken 4-6 weeks apart.

Ref: NICE Guidelines NG23 –Menopause: Diagnosis and management

104. B

Common unwanted outcome after endometrial ablation are vaginal discharge, increased period pain or cramping and need for additional surgery.

Ref: NICE Guidelines CG44 – Heavy menstrual bleeding: assessment and management

105. A

Retinoids are absolute contraindication during pregnancy and at least 2 years before.

Ref: BASHH Guidelines- UK National Guideline on the Management of Vulval conditions.

106. A

Prophylactic vaginal progesterone should be given to women with no history of preterm birth or mid-trimester loss with cervical length of less than 25mm between 16 and 24 weeks gestation

Ref: NICE Guidelines NG25 –Preterm Labour and Birth

107. B

To identify infection in women with PPROM use a combination of clinical assessment and tests (CRP, WBC and measurement of fetal heart rate using CTG to diagnose intrauterine infection.

Ref: NICE Guidelines NG25 –Preterm Labour and Birth

108. D

Ref: NICE Guidelines NG3 – Diabetes in pregnancy: management from preconception to the postnatal period

109. C

If sepsis is suspected in the community, urgent referral to hospital is indicated if there are red flag signs and symptoms

Ref: Bacterial sepsis following pregnancy
Green-top Guideline No. 64b

110. A

Ref: Bacterial sepsis following pregnancy
Green-top Guideline No. 64b

111. C

Ref: Bacterial sepsis following pregnancy
Green-top Guideline No. 64b

112. B

Ref: Chicken pox in pregnancy
Green-top Guideline No. 13

113. D

Ref: BASHH Guidelines: Management of Genital Herpes in pregnancy

114. C

Ref: BASHH Guidelines: Management of Genital Herpes in pregnancy

115. C

Ref: The management of sexually transmitted infections in pregnancy
TOG 2012, Volume 14, 1

116. D

Relative contraindications where ECV might be more complicated:

- Small-for-gestational-age fetus with abnormal Doppler parameters
- Proteinuric pre-eclampsia
- Oligohydramnios
- Major fetal anomalies
- Scarred uterus (previous Caesarean section)
- Unstable lie.

Ref: External cephalic version (ECV) and reducing the incidence of breech presentation
RCOG Green-top Guideline No. 20 a

117. B

One of the principal concerns of diabetic pregnancy is the risk of congenital malformations, most common seen are neural tube defects, congenital heart disease, malformations of renal and urinary tract gastrointestinal and skeletal malformations

Nelson–Piercy C. Handbook of Obstetric Medicine, 4th. London: Informa Healthcare, 2010

118. B

Ref: Shoulder Dystocia
Green-top Guideline No. 42

119. B

While the use of the patient's relatives or friends may sometimes be useful in urgent cases, it is preferable to ensure that the patient have an unbiased interpretation of the doctor's explanation.

Ref: Obtaining valid consent
Clinical governance advice no.6

120. B

While the use of the patient's relatives or friends may sometimes be useful in urgent cases, it is preferable to ensure that the patient have an unbiased interpretation of the doctor's explanation.

Ref: Obtaining valid consent
Clinical governance advice no.6

121. D

When performing surgery in women with ovarian endometrioma, ovarian cystectomy should be performed as it reduces endometriosis -associated pain.

Ref: Management of women with endometriosis

Guideline of the European society of human reproduction and embryology 2013

122. B

Physiological changes of pregnancy increase level of thyroid -binding globulin in response to oestrogen stimulation coupled with reduced clearance of thyroxine-binding globulin and increased glomerular filtration rate increasing clearance of free thyroid hormones.

Ref: Thyroid dysfunction and reproductive health

TOG 2015, Volume 17, 1

123. C

Ref: Thyroid dysfunction and reproductive health

TOG 2015, Volume 16, 1

124. D

A migraine is classically unilateral, pulsating and builds over minutes to hours and moderate to severe in intensity and associated with nausea and vomiting and is aggravated by routine physical activity

Ref: Headache in pregnancy

TOG 2014, Volume 16, 3

125. A

Ref: Headache in pregnancy

TOG 2014, Volume 16, 3

126. C

Magnetic resonance venography is the imaging modality of choice.

Ref: Headache in pregnancy

TOG 2014, Volume 16, 3

127. A

Ref: Headache in pregnancy

TOG 2014, Volume 16, 3

128. E

Ref: Headache in pregnancy
TOG 2014, Volume 16, 3

129. D

Elective delivery by caesarean section in asymptomatic women is not recommended before 38weeks of gestation for placenta praevia, or before 36-37 weeks of gestation for suspected placenta accrete

Ref: Placenta praevia, placenta praevia accreta and Vasa praevia: Diagnosis and Management
Green-top Guideline No. 27

130. D

15% of cases the vasa praevia can resolve in hence imaging should be repeated in the third trimester to confirm persistence.
Ref: Placenta praevia, placenta praevia accreta and Vasa praevia: Diagnosis and Management
Green-top Guideline No. 27

131. C

15% of cases the vasa praevia can resolve.
Ref: Placenta praevia, placenta praevia accreta and Vasa praevia: Diagnosis and Management
Green-top Guideline No. 27

132. C 35 - 37 wks

Ref: Placenta praevia, placenta praevia accreta and Vasa praevia: Diagnosis and Management
Green-top Guideline No. 27

133. C ? B

Anti -K antibodies referral should take place once detected, as severe anaemia can occur even with low titre
Ref: The management of women with red cell antibodies during pregnancy
Green-top Guideline No. 65

134. B

Referral to fetal medicine should be made once anti-c levels are>7.5iu/ml as this correlates with a moderate risk of HDFN.

Ref: The management of women with red cell antibodies during pregnancy Green-top Guideline No. 65

135. A

	OC Present	OC Absent
Test Positive	70 (True positive)	345 (False positive)
Test Negative	40 (False negative)	1345 (True negative)

False Positive Rate = 1 – specificity = FP/(FP+TN) = 345/(345+1345)

Ref: Statistical Analysis

136. B

	OC Present	OC Absent
Test Positive	70 (True positive)	345 (False positive)
Test Negative	40 (False negative)	1345 (True negative)

False Negative Rate = 1- sensitivity = FN/(TP+ FN) = 40/(70+40)

Ref: Statistical Analysis

137. A

Clinical Governance

Ref: RCOG Clinical Governance Papers

138. C

Non -immune pregnant women who have been exposed to chicken pox should be managed as potentially infectious from day 8-28 days after exposure if they receive VZIG and from day 8-21 days after exposure if they do not receive VZIG.

Ref: Chicken pox in pregnancy Green-top Guideline No. 13

139. E

Oral aciclovir should be prescribed for pregnant women with chicken pox if they present within 24 hours of onset of the rash and if they are 20 weeks of gestation or beyond. IV aciclovir should be given to all pregnant women with severe chicken pox.

Ref: Chicken pox in pregnancy
Green-top Guideline No. 13

140. C

In a febrile patient, three negative malaria smears 12-24 hours apart rules out the diagnosis of malaria.

Ref: The diagnosis and treatment malaria in pregnancy.
Green-top Guideline No. 54B

141. C

Ref: Monochorionic Twin pregnancy, Management.
Green-top Guideline No. 51

142. C

Ref: Monochorionic Twin pregnancy, Management.
Green-top Guideline No. 51

143. D

MRI has a sensitivity of 91% and a specificity of 98% with avoidance of exposure to radiation

Ref: Appendicitis in pregnancy: how to manage and whether to deliver
TOG 2015, Volume 17, 2

144. C

Ref: Caesarean Section for Placenta Praevia
RCOG Consent Advice No. 12

145. D

Most sensitive and specific marker is ST elevation, which normally appears within a few minutes of onset of symptoms.

Ref: Myocardial infarction and pregnancy
TOG 2013, Volume 15, 4

146. B

Postpartum psychosis is a psychiatric emergency; the clinical picture may mislead, quickly become extremely severe and vary significantly from hour to hour. Admission is usually necessary even for women with the most supportive of families.

Ref: Postpartum psychosis
TOG 2013, Volume 15, 3

147. D

Treatment should not be delayed and should be in line with her clinical condition

Ref: BASHH Guidelines: Management of Genital Herpes in pregnancy

148. C

GBS bacteriuria is associated with a higher risk of chorioamnionitis and neonatal disease hence GBS bacteriuria during pregnancy should receive appropriate treatment at time of diagnosis as well as IAP.

Ref: The prevention of early-onset neonatal group B streptococcal disease.
Green-top Guideline No. 36

149. D

Iron chelators should be reviewed and deferasirox and deferiprone ideally discontinued 3 months before conception. Desferrioxamine should be avoided in the first trimester due to lack of safety data. HbA1c is not a reliable marker of glycaemic control as this is diluted by transfused blood and results in underestimation.

Ref: Management of Beta Thalassaemia in pregnancy.
Green-top Guideline No. 66

150. B

Consider prophylactic cervical cerclage for women in whom TVS reveal cervical length of less than25mm and who have either had history of preterm prelabour rupture of membranes.

Ref: NICE Guidelines NG25 –Preterm Labour and Birth

151. E

Live vaccines are generally contraindicated in pregnancy

Ref: Vaccination in pregnancy
TOG 2015, Volume 17, 4

152. C

Women with Thalassaemia who have undergone splenectomy or have a platelet count greater than 600 X 10^9/l should have low-dose aspirin but if they have both then should be offered low-molecular weight heparin thromboprophylaxis as well as low dose aspirin. They also need thromboprophylaxis during antenatal hospital admissions.

Ref: Management of Beta Thalassaemia in pregnancy.
Green-top Guideline No. 66

153. C

Ref: Nice guideline on antenatal and postnatal mental health (CG 192)

154. E

Affects about 1in 1000 in post partum, valproate is associated with fetal anomalies and neurodevelopmental problems.

Ref: Nice guideline on antenatal and postnatal mental health (CG 192)

155. A

Lithium should be stopped gradually over about 4 weeks; risk of fetal cardiac anomalies may not be reduced when it is stopped. If this is the only medication working for the patient or risks relapse if stopped, consider stopping and restarting in second trimester.

Ref: Nice guideline on antenatal and postnatal mental health (CG 192)

156. A

The NICE guideline recommends that such women deliver not later than 40 weeks and 6 days, offering induction at 40 weeks and 4 days therefore is reasonable. Steroids is only required if she is going to be delivered by caesarean section

Ref: NICE CG: NG3, Diabetes in pregnancy

157. D

She needs yearly fasting plasma glucose 6 to13 weeks postnatal and yearly plasma glucose if the fasting plasma glucose is normal and advice on lifestyle changes (diet and exercise)

Ref: NICE CG: NG3, Diabetes in pregnancy

158. D

The only indication for GTT is diabetes in first pregnancy even if they had a pregnancy without diabetes. Routinely GTT may be part of the antenatal screening in high-risk population areas.

Ref: NICE CG: NG3, Diabetes in pregnancy

159. C

Capillary glucose is monitored every hour ensuring it is maintained between 4 and 7mmol/l. Sliding scale with dextrose and insulin should be used if this is not maintained between 4 and 7mmol/l.

Ref: NICE CG: NG3, Diabetes in pregnancy

160. A

Ref: RCOG GTG: 55: Late Intrauterine Fetal Death and Stillbirth

161. E

The rest are all associated with intrauterine fetal death

Ref: RCOG GTG: 55: Late Intrauterine Fetal Death and Stillbirth

162. B

This percentage may vary but less than 10% and more that 2%.

Ref: RCOG GTG: 55: Late Intrauterine Fetal Death and Stillbirth

163. A

Prostaglandins with mifepristone are recommended as the first line method but misoprostol is cheaper and has similar efficacy and safety profile.

Ref: RCOG GTG: 55: Late Intrauterine Fetal Death and Stillbirth

164. B

As this is an intrauterine fetal death, she does not require prophylaxis for GBS, Ciprofloxacin is the first line antibiotics for UTI. She will require broad-spectrum antibiotics if sepsis is suspected.

165. C

Recession of the fetal head during labour should raise suspicion of a scar dehiscence or rupture. Haematuria rather than Anuria is a likely sign.

Ref: RCOG GTG 45: Birth after Previous Caesarean Birth

166. D

Congenital heart defects especially Patent Ductus Arteriosus (PDA) is a feature of congenital rubella but not the other options. All the other features are present in all the other options.

167. B

Initial first line management involves rest, hydration, simple analgesia, anti-emetics and avoiding precipitating factors. The risk of pre-eclampsia is more than 2 times and not 5 times and the risk of stroke is higher than the risk of myocardial infarction.

Ref: TOG, Vol 16. No 3 2014

168. B

Ref: TOG Vol 16, no 3, and 2014

169. E

A large bore cannula, a 16 or 14-gauge cannula should be used. Prophylactic Oxytocics reduce PPH by 60%. Carbetocin is licensed in the UK for prevention of PPH in caesarean sections.

Ref: RCOG GTG: 52: Prevention and Management of Postpartum Haemorrhage

170. D

With women on cART and very low (undetectable viral load) the Mother to child transmission rate is about 0.57%

BHIVA Guidelines for management of HIV infection in pregnant women: 2012

171. A

There are a small proportion of HIV positive people who will have undetectable VL (on two different assays) known as Elite controllers. Pregnant women in this group should be treated with cART or monotherapy with zidovudine. Monotherapy with other agents is not recommended and the woman is advised to exclusively formula feed. There is no evidence that cART is superior to zidovudine alone in reducing vaginal shedding hence zidovudine monotherapy is an acceptable choice.

BHIVA Guidelines for management of HIV infection in pregnant women: 2012

172. D

This is also known as Group A beta haemolytic streptococci

Ref: RCOG Guideline on sepsis following pregnancy: GTG: 64b

173. C

The risk in subsequent pregnancies is 5-7%. The overall incidence of AOSIS is 2.9%, 6.1% in primips and 1.7% in multips

Ref: RCOG GTG 29: Management of third and fourth degree perineal tears: 2015

174. E

Risk of placenta previa is 1% after one caesarean section and 1.7% after 2 from a systematic review. The risk of scar dehiscence is about 0.5% and 1.4% after 1 and 2 previous caesarean sections respectively. The risk of birth related perinatal death is almost the same

Ref: RCOG GTG: 45: Birth after Previous Caesarean Birth: 2015

175. C

There is significant difference in the other options

Ref: NICE Intrapartum care for healthy women and babies: CG190

176. D

Ref: RCOG GTG 26: Operative Vaginal Delivery: 2011

177. B

Air travel is allowed till 36 weeks in an uncomplicated singleton pregnancy and till 32 weeks in an uncomplicated multiple pregnancies.

Ref: Air Travel In Pregnancy
Scientific Impact Paper No. 1

178. C

There are some contraindications to air travel if there is associated medical problems such as severe anemia <7.5g/dl, recent hemorrhage, otitis media and sinusitis, serious cardiac and respiratory disease, recent sickling crisis, recent gastrointestinal surgery, a fracture where significant leg swelling can occur in flight.

Ref: Air Travel In Pregnancy
Scientific Impact Paper No. 1

179. C

Fetal scalp lactate has been found to be better tool in predicting hypoxic ischemic encephalopathy in a fetus compared to fetal scalp pH. Lactate levels <4.2 is normal and labour should be allowed to continue. If the Lactate levels

are 4.2 – 4.8, repeat FBS should be done in 20 – 30 mins. If the lactate level >4.8 – delivery should be considered.
Ref: Is it Time for UK Obstetricians to Accept Fetal Scalp Lactate as an Alternative to Scalp pH?
Scientific Impact Paper No. 47

180. B

The risk of stillbirth is higher in women ≥ 40. It is 2 in 1000 at 39 – 40 weeks compared to 1 in 1000 for women <35 years of age.
Ref: Induction of Labour at Term in Older Mothers
Scientific Impact Paper No. 34

181. B

Risk of primary caesarean section is high with hypovitaminosis D. The other risks are preeclampsia, hypertension, low birthweight of the baby, bacterial vaginosis in the mother, fetal wheeze and asthma and neonatal hypocalcemia.
Ref: Vitamin D In Pregnancy
Scientific Paper No: 43

182. A

The centre of ventouse cup should be placed on the flexion point so that traction in the line of pelvic axis will result in most flexed suboccipitobregmatic diameter. The flexion point is 3cm on the sagittal suture in front of the posterior fontanelle.
Ref: Management of Delivery when malposition of the fetal head complicates the second stage of labour
TOG 2015, Volume 17,4

183. B

Remifentanil is a rapidly acting synthetic opioid with a half-life of 3 minutes. It takes 5 minutes to work. 1 in 8 women may need additional Entonox. It is safe for the fetus and continuous fetal monitoring is not required. Oxygen saturation monitoring is required but blood pressure monitoring is not needed. The failure rate is same as epidural at 1 in 10.
Ref: Analgesia for labour: An evidence based insight for the obstetrician
TOG 2015, Volume 17, 3

184. D

Prophylaxis is not needed if elective caesarean section or if GBS screen was positive in previous pregnancy but the baby did not have early onset GBS

infection. Prophylaxis should be given if there is significant GBS bacteriuria (>10^5 cfs/ml). It is also not indicated in preterm rupture of membrane unless there are signs of infection. It is indicated if GBS is incidentally picked up antenatally during vaginal swab for any other reason.
Ref: RCOG GTG No. 36: Prevention of Early Onset Neonatal GBS

185. D
Ref: RCOG GTG No. 51: Management of Monochorionic twin pregnancy

186. D
Alkaline phosphatase is increased in cholestasis but not helpful in diagnosis since in pregnancy it is mostly placental in origin. Both conjugated and unconjugated bilirubin may increase in Obstetric cholestasis (intrahepatic)
Ref: RCOG GTG No.43:Obstetrics Cholestasis

187. C
With major low lying placenta or those with previous caesarean section, a repeat ultrasound scan is suggested at 32weeks; for minor placenta praevia 36 weeks will suffice. A transvaginal scan (along with transabdominal) is necessary to diagnose. MRI is not needed routinely to exclude placenta accreta – it is needed where there is doubt after ultrasound
Placenta Praevia, Placenta Praevia Accreta and Vasa Praevia: Diagnosis and Management
Ref: RCOG GTG No.27

188. C
Oxytocin is the first line prophylaxis for low risk delivery: IM for vaginal and IV for caesarean section. Syntometrine is the first line unless hypertensive: in high risk eg. Anaemia. Misoprostol 600 mcg orally is not as effective but is the second line if oxytocin is not available. Carbetocin is not yet recommended.
Ref: Prevention and Management of postpartum haemorrhage
RCOG GTG No. 52

189. D
Nifedipine is better than beta agonists in delaying labour and improving neonatal outcome and is comparable to atosiban (oxytocin receptor agonist) but is not licensed in the U.K. for this indication.
Ref: RCOG GTG No.18: Tocolysis for women in preterm labour

190. C

CVS should be performed after 10 weeks. Risk of oromandibular limb hypoplasia and difficulty in performing are minimised after 10 weeks. Early amniocentesis (before 14 weeks) is associated with talipes, miscarriage and respiratory problems. Amniocentesis in the 3rd trimester is not associated with any increased risk of emergency delivery. There is a greater likelihood of multiple attempts and blood stained fluid in the 3rd trimester as compared to the 2nd trimester. Amniocentesis can be done in Hepatitis B or C carriers so long as they are appropriately counselled.

Ref: RCOG GTG No.8: Amniocentesis and Chorionic Villus Sampling

191. B

In intrauterine growth restriction steroids are given between 24 and 35+6weeks gestation. In the case of multiple pregnancies or any women where there is a higher risk of preterm labour, it should be given upto 34+6 weeks. Even in overt chorioamnionitis steroids can be given but this should not delay delivery. Most robust data is from 26 weeks onward.

Ref: RCOG GTG No.7: Antenatal corticosteroids to reduce neonatal mortality and morbidity

192. A

There is no evidence to suggest formal foetal count monitoring (foetal kick chart). All others are valid investigations. Visual or computerised assessments of CTG are both acceptable. Even though there is no evidence to recommend biophysical profile, in selected high-risk cases it may have a role.

Ref: RCOG GTG No. 57: Reduced Foetal Movement

193. E

Amniocentesis is not contraindicated even if alloimmunisation has occurred. Refer to FMU if Anti D titres > 4 IU/ml, Anti c > 7.5 IU/ml and presence of any Anti K antibodies. Anti E if present along with Anti c potentiates the foetal anaemia and therefore should be referred to FMU (not if alone).

Ref: RCOG GTG No. 65: The Management of Women with Red Cell Antibodies in Pregnancy

194. B

In cell salvage and reinfusion, a minimum of 1500 IU/ml of Anti D Immunoglobulin should be administered once cord blood confirms D positive.

Also 30-45 minutes after reinfusion, Kleihauer should be done to see if additional Anti D is needed.
Ref: BCSH guideline for the use of Anti D immunoglobulin for the prevention of haemolytic disease of the foetus and newborn

195. B

Group A Streptococcus should be suspected if the woman presents within 12 hours of delivery. Severe pain in the limbs in sepsis is likely to be an early sign of Necrotising fasciitis or myositis. She is obviously in septic shock, therefore, Intensivist, microbiologist should be involved at the earliest and transfer to ITU considered. Surgical referral should ideally be to Plastic surgeon for necrotising fasciitis. Newborn should be treated irrespective of whether there are clinical signs of infection in the newborn or not. Analgesics should be given but NSAID should be avoided since NSAID s impede the ability of the polymorphs to fight Group A streptococcus infection.
Ref: RCOG GTG No. 64B: Bacterial Sepsis Following Pregnancy

196. A

The leading indirect cause of death in the last MBRRACE report is cardiac disease as it has been previously. Thrombosis and thromboembolism are the leading direct cause of death.
Ref: MBRRACE UK Update
TOG 2016, Vol 18, 1

197. B

Initiation of Breast-feeding is delayed in women with spinal cord injury above T4. This is because milk ejection reflex is initiated by infant suckling and is carried from the tactile receptors of the breast via the dorsal roots of T4 – T6. These women need support in the form of visual stimulation or oxytocin nasal spray. Long-term breastfeeding is maintained. Autonomic dysreflexia is rare in breastfeeding.
Ref: Pregnancy and Spinal Cord Injury
TOG 2014; Vol 16, 2

198. C

When the CTG has 1 abnormal feature, it needs further testing. If the FBS fails, but there is acceleration on fetal scalp stimulation, it is likely that the baby is not decompensating. It should be discussed with Consultant Obstetrician (in this case, the FBS was attempted by the resident consultant) and upon discussion with the mother; labour can be continued if the CTG does

not deteriorate. In this case, the mother is committed to vaginal delivery. So labour can continue until the CTG worsens.
Ref: Intrapartum Care For Healthy Women and Babies
NICE Guideline CG190

199. B

Formative OSATs should be used for supervised learning event. This gives an opportunity for practising and receiving feedback. Summative OSATs should be used for assessment of performance. This is to demonstrate competence and progress in training.
Ref: RCOG Careers and Training – Work placed based assessment tools

200. B

The risk of laceration to bladder, bowel and uterine extension is in the range of 10% to 27%
Ref: Caesarean section at full dilatation: incidence, impact and current management
TOG 2014; Vol 16, 3

About the Authors

Sharmistha Guha MRCOG, PG Cert (Gynae Ultrasound) is a Consultant Obstetrician & Gynaecologist at West Middlesex University Hospital, London. She has done advanced training in Acute Gynaecology and Early Pregnancy Care, Gynaecological Ultrasound, Benign Open and Laparoscopic Gynaecological Surgery and Advanced Labour Ward Practice. She has been the co- lead for the London SBA Writing Group for the RCOG and has contributed questions to the RCOG Question Bank and the RCOG SBA book. She has organized and taught in MRCOG Part 2 theory and OSCE Courses for the London Deanery and in India. She has several publications in peer reviewed journals and has reviewed chapters in books and papers for prestigious journals. She has presented in many national and international conferences and is the ATSM Preceptor for Acute Gynaecology and Early Pregnancy in Northwest London.

Parijat Bhattacharjee MRCOG is a Consultant Obstetrician and Gynaecologist at the London North West NHS Trust. He is actively involved in teaching undergraduate medical students from Imperial College School of Medicine, London and teaches in the Enhanced Revision Programme for MRCOG Part 2 examinations of the Royal College of Obstetrician and Gynaecologist. He is also actively involved in Obstetrics & Gynaecology training and workshops in Africa and Asia. His clinical and research interests are Infertility and Minimal Access Surgery.

Nutan Mishra MD, FRCOG is a Consultant in Obstetrician and Gynaecologist at Buckinghamshire Healthcare NHS Trust. Her main interests are high risk pregnancy, particularly pre-eclampsia and diabetes and fetal growth restriction. She is actively involved in teaching and training and is the medical student coordinator for the Oxford rotation. She is a facilitator for the RCOG Basic Surgical Skills Course, MRCOG OCSE and CTG training courses. She has written book chapters on Postpartum haemorrhage and Uterine rupture and facilitates courses on Basic Emergency Obstetric care and Newborn care.

Francis Ayim MRCOG is a Consultant Obstetrician & Gynaecologist at Hillingdon Hospital NHS Trust. His special interests are Early Pregnancy Care, Emergency and Ambulatory Gynaecology and Obstetrics. He is a facilitator for the RCOG Hysteroscopy Course and teaches on Communication skills and consultant preparation courses.

INDEX

B

C

D

E

I

J

K

L

M

N

O

P

T

U

V

W

Y